CASE REVIEW

Obstetric and Gynecologic Ultrasound

Series Editor

David M. Yousem, MD
Professor, Department of Radiology and Radiological Sciences
Director of Neuroradiology
Johns Hopkins Hospital
Baltimore, Maryland

Other Volumes in the CASE REVIEW Series

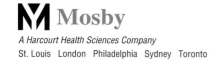

A Harcourt Health Sciences Company
St. Louis London Philadelphia Sydney Toronto

Pamela T. Johnson, MD
Assistant Professor
Department of Radiology
Thomas Jefferson University Hospital
Philadelphia, Pennsylvania

Alfred B. Kurtz, MD
Professor and Vice Chairman
Department of Radiology
Thomas Jefferson University Hospital
Philadelphia, Pennsylvania

CASE REVIEW

Obstetric and Gynecologic Ultrasound

CASE REVIEW SERIES

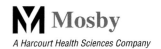

A Harcourt Health Sciences Company

Editor-in-Chief: Richard Lampert
Acquisitions Editor: Stephanie Donley
Manuscript Editor: Marjory I. Fraser
Production Manager: Frank Polizzano
Illustration Specialist: Rita Martello
Book Designer: Gene Harris
Indexer: Angela M. Holt

Copyright © 2001 by Mosby, Inc.

Mosby, Inc.
A Harcourt Health Sciences Company
11830 Westline Industrial Drive
St. Louis, Missouri 63146

Printed in the United States of America

Library of Congress Cataloging-in-Publication Data

Johnson, Pamela Teece.
Obsterics and gynecologic ultrasound: case review/Pamela Teece Johnson, Alfred B. Kurtz.—1st ed.

p. cm.

ISBN 0–323–00860–7

1. Generative organs, Female—Ultrasonic imaging.
    2. Fetus—Diseases—Diagnosis.   3. Ultrasonics in obstetrics.
    I. Kurtz, Alfred B.   II. Title

RG107.5.U4 J647 2001
618'.047543—dc21   2001030419

01 02 03 04 05 WBS/MP 9   8   7   6   5   4   3   2   1

To the radiology residents, whose quest for knowledge inspired this book.

If radiologists are to maintain their pre-eminent role in obstetric and gynecologic ultrasound, we must strive for excellence in the field. In the current milieu of innumerable turf wars and encroachment of nonradiologists on imaging studies, the only principle that we can fall back on is the strength of our patient service and the quality of our interpretations. Obstetric ultrasound is a very difficult technique to conquer, and the stakes of potential errors in interpretation can be enormous. Gynecologic sonograms have become one of the most common studies requested in busy urban emergency rooms, and the findings may often precipitate surgical interventions.

In this volume of the Case Review series, Drs Johnson and Kurtz have selected an outstanding array of cases that teach the reader the intricacies of mastering obstetric and gynecologic ultrasound. Their accompanying text includes many pertinent references as well as tricks of the trade to guide the practitioner.

The Case Review series is designed to review each specialty in a challenging interactive way. Each book in the series has gradations of difficulty so that the reader can assess his or her proficiency and can use this self-evaluation to guide continued education. By referencing THE REQUISITES series, the reader can obtain "ultrasonic feedback" if a weakness is perceived. Because each case is distinct, this is the kind of textbook that can be picked up and read at any time of day in your career.

I am very pleased to have Drs Johnson and Kurtz's edition join the ever-expanding Case Review series. I welcome the *Obstetric and Gynecologic Ultrasound: Case Review* to the previously published volumes on *Thoracic Imaging* by Phil Boiselle and Theresa McLoud; *Genitourinary Imaging* by Glenn Tung, Ron Zagoria, and William Mayo-Smith; *Gastrointestinal Imaging* by Peter Feczko and Robert Halpert; *Brain Imaging* by Laurie Loevner; and *Head and Neck Imaging* by myself. Congratulations.

David M. Yousem, MD

This case review series focuses on ultrasound in obstetrics and gynecology. We would like to recognize the important accomplishments of Dr. Barry Goldberg, whose leadership and unique abilities have created one of the strongest ultrasound laboratories in the world. He has forged and maintained strong relationships with other disciplines in all fields of medicine. This has allowed us, as radiologists and sonologists, to have the opportunity of working and interacting with excellent obstetricians, gynecologists, and perinatologists. This cooperation has led to high-quality care for patients and serves as the case material for this book.

Our goals in writing this book were two-fold. The first goal was to compile what we believed was a comprehensive list of entities in obstetric and gynecologic ultrasound. We then searched diligently to find the best example of each entity, occasionally relying on invaluable contributions from outside contributors. The second goal was to illustrate and discuss the ultrasound findings for each diagnosis, incorporating data from the latest radiology and obstetrics literature. Because the field of obstetric and gynecologic ultrasonography continues to grow, we reviewed all pertinent literature within the text of each case. Although this case review series is designed to prepare residents and fellows for an oral board-type examination, we hope that this approach will also serve as a review for any physician who performs obstetric and gynecologic imaging.

We thank all of those who contributed or assisted in obtaining cases, including Dr. Beryl Benacerraf, Dr. George Bega, Dr. Anna Lev-Toaff, Dr. Beverly Coleman, Dr. Mary C. Frates, Ms. Anita Urban, Ms. Katie James, and especially Mr. Dennis Woods who provided most of the cardiac cases. Our photography experts, Mr. Fred Ross and Mr. Ken Goodman, played an integral part in the preparation of the images. Finally, we would like to thank our department chairman, Dr. David Levin, for his support and understanding and for creating the academic atmosphere within which such projects can flourish.

Opening Round

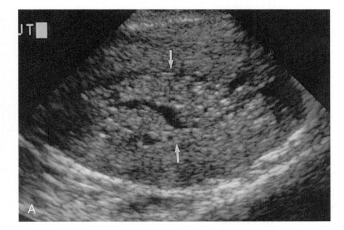

1. A 60-year-old woman on long-term treatment with tamoxifen presents with a transvaginal sagittal image of the uterus (Fig. A: arrows = endometrial thickness of 14 mm). Is this considered to be normal?
2. What is the effect of tamoxifen on the uterus?
3. What is the spectrum of endometrial abnormalities that tamoxifen induces?
4. What is the cutoff for an abnormal endometrial thickness in a woman taking tamoxifen?

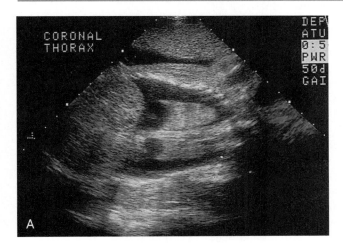

1. In this third-trimester fetus, what is the finding on this coronal image of the fetal chest (Fig. A)?
2. What are the potential complications?
3. What is the outcome?
4. What is the treatment if this persists or recurs?

Tamoxifen

1. No, this is diffuse endometrial thickening and may be benign but cannot be considered to be normal.

2. Estrogenic.

3. Endometrial hyperplasia, endometrial and endocervical polyps, subendometrial cysts, and endometrial cancer.

4. 8 mm or greater.

References

Hann LE, Giess CS, Bach AM, et al: Endometrial thickness in tamoxifen-treated patients: Correlation with clinical and pathologic findings. *AJR Am J Roentgenol* 168:657–661, 1997.

Hulka CA, Hall DA: Endometrial abnormalities associated with tamoxifen therapy for breast cancer: Sonographic and pathologic correlation. *AJR Am J Roentgenol* 160:809–812, 1993.

Cross-Reference

Ultrasound: THE REQUISITES, pp 368–374.

Comment

Tamoxifen is a widely used medication for patients with breast cancer, because of the antiestrogenic effect on breast tissue. However, the medication can have an estrogenic effect on the endometrium. Accordingly, these women are predisposed to develop a number of different endometrial abnormalities, including polyps of the endometrium and endocervix, subendometrial cysts, endometrial hyperplasia, and cancer. The risk of developing one of these endometrial pathologies relates to the duration of tamoxifen therapy; the most common abnormality is an endometrial polyp.

Ultrasound is an excellent screening tool to detect endometrial abnormalities, by demonstrating an endometrial thickness of more than 8 mm. Endometrial thickening 8 mm or greater warrants biopsy. A hyperechoic endometrium with small cystic spaces is the classic finding associated with tamoxifen therapy (see Fig. A). Many of these represent endometrial polyps; however, more than one pathologic process (e.g., hyperplasia) may be present.

One study demonstrated that most women on tamoxifen *do not* have symptoms such as bleeding. Nonetheless, almost half of these women had abnormal endometrial thickness on ultrasound (defined as >8 mm). Although the risk may be increased as much as 6-fold, fewer than 1% of the women taking tamoxifen therapy develop endometrial cancer. Most of *these* women have been receiving the treatment for more than 5 years, and most present with postmenopausal bleeding.

Notes

Pleural Effusions

1. Bilateral pleural effusions.

2. Inhibition of pulmonary development, hydrops, and polyhydramnios.

3. Variable from normal to fetal death.

4. Thoracocentesis and thoracoamniotic shunt if large and recurrent.

Acknowledgment

Figure for Case 2 courtesy of Mr. Dennis Woods.

References

Achiron R, Weissman A, Lipitz S, et al: Fetal pleural effusion: The risk of fetal trisomy. *Gynecol Obstet Invest* 39:153–156, 1995.

Ahmad FK, Sherman SJ, Hagglund KH, et al: Isolated unilateral fetal pleural effusion: The role of sonographic surveillance and in utero therapy. *Fetal Diagn Ther* 11:383–389, 1996.

Cross-Reference

Ultrasound: THE REQUISITES, pp 249–250.

Comment

Fetal pleural effusion can present in the first, second, or third trimester. Ultrasound demonstrates fluid surrounding the lungs, which can have a "batwing" appearance when bilateral, as shown in this case. There are a number of possible causes, including chylothorax, chromosomal anomalies, cardiac malformations, infection, pulmonary lymphangiectasia, pulmonary mass, and hydrops fetalis in conjunction with accumulation of fluid elsewhere and thickening of the skin.

Karyotyping is advised whether or not additional malformations are present to suggest a chromosomal anomaly. Isolated pleural effusion has been associated with trisomy 21 and Turner's syndrome and detected as early as the first trimester. The incidence of such a chromosomal anomaly is as high as 6%.

The course of fetal pleural effusion is variable. Almost 10% of small effusions can resolve spontaneously. If thoracocentesis is performed before delivery, some cases will not reaccumulate, and one lung can expand when the newborn attempts to breathe. However, small effusions can grow rapidly, with risk of secondary polyhydramnios, nonimmune hydrops, and underdevelopment of the compressed lung. Thus, careful follow-up ultrasound, as frequently as twice a week, has been recommended. If a large volume of fluid reaccumulates, a thoracoamniotic shunt can be placed to improve the outcome.

Notes

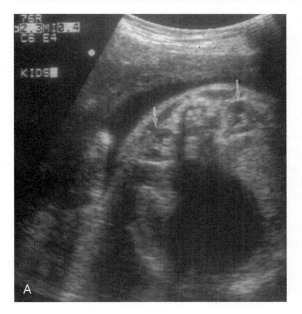

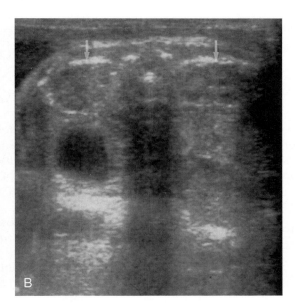

1. What is the location of the cystic abnormalities shown in these axial images of the fetal abdomen in these two third-trimester fetuses (Figs. A and B, both at the level of the kidneys denoted by arrows)?

2. Name the type of fetal abdominal mass that can have both cystic and solid components.

3. Which cystic mass may have internal echoes?

4. Which associated anomalies may be seen with enteric duplication cysts?

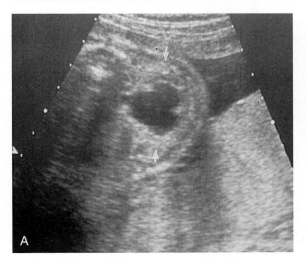

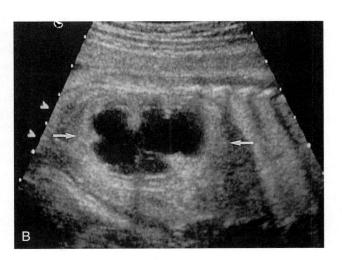

1. In this early third-trimester fetus, what do the axial (Fig. A) and sagittal (Fig. B) images detect in a fetal kidney (arrows)?

2. What is the most common cause of hydronephrosis in the neonate?

3. What is the incidence of contralateral renal abnormalities with this entity?

4. Are extrarenal anomalies associated?

CASE 3

Cystic Abdominal Mass

1. Intra-abdominal (not retroperitoneal).

2. Teratomas, either ovarian or retroperitoneal.

3. Meconium pseudocyst.

4. Spinal or gastrointestinal malformations.

References

Foster MA, Nyberg DA, Mahoney BS, et al: Meconium peritonitis: Prenatal sonographic findings and their clinical significance. *Radiology* 165:661–665, 1987.

Richards DS, Langham MR, Anderson CD: The prenatal sonographic appearance of enteric duplication cysts. *Ultrasound Obstet Gynecol* 7:17–20, 1996.

Cross-Reference
Ultrasound: THE REQUISITES, pp 269–271.

Comment

The differential list for a cystic abdominal or pelvic mass in a fetus is long. Identification of associated findings may aid in determining the precise etiology. In these two cases, the cystic masses do not extend back to the spine and are not related to the kidneys so that renal and retroperitoneal masses do not need to be considered.

Ovarian cysts are among the most common cystic abdominal masses in females. Simple cysts (see Fig. A) and teratomas can arise from the ovary. Obstruction of the vagina or uterus may appear as a cystic mass in the pelvic midline.

A simple cyst may represent a mesenteric or omental cyst; additionally, enteric duplication cysts are located in the mesentery. Enteric duplication cysts (see Fig. B) are directly contiguous with the bowel and may communicate with the bowel lumen. Approximately 30% of fetuses with enteric duplication cysts have associated anomalies. Spinal or gastrointestinal malformations may be present with foregut or hindgut duplications, respectively.

A meconium pseudocyst forms from walled-off complicated ascites secondary to meconium peritonitis. The cyst typically contains internal echoes. Dilatation of the small bowel, peritoneal calcifications, and polyhydramnios can be seen. The obstructed bowel loop in bowel atresia can also present as an abdominal cystic mass, usually with hyperperistalsis.

Genitourinary cysts can arise from several sites. Renal causes such as multicystic dysplastic kidney have been eliminated in this case. However, posterior urethral valve (PUV) obstruction can result in urinoma formation. An obstructed bladder in PUV or other types of bladder outlet obstruction appear as large cystic pelvic-abdominal masses. The existence of a urachal cyst is an additional possibility.

Notes

CASE 4

Ureteropelvic Junction Obstruction

1. Hydronephrosis.

2. Ureteropelvic junction (UPJ) obstruction.

3. 20%.

4. Yes.

Reference

Bosman G, Reuss A, Nijman M, Wladimiroff JW: Prenatal diagnosis, management and outcome of fetal ureteropelvic junction obstruction. *Ultrasound Med Biol* 17:117–120, 1991.

Cross-Reference
Ultrasound: THE REQUISITES, pp 283–285.

Comment

UPJ obstruction is the most common cause of hydronephrosis in the neonate. The cause is considered to be an intrinsic functional obstruction of outflow from the renal pelvis owing to abnormal development. Infrequently, an obstructing vessel or other anatomic cause is implicated.

On prenatal ultrasound, dilatation of the renal pelvis is seen. The degree of dilatation has been classified using ultrasound, depending on the pelvic diameter (<1 cm, 1 to 1.5 cm, >1 cm) and the presence and degree of caliectasis (none, moderate, or marked). Once dilatation has been detected, postnatal follow-up is essential to determine the degree of residual renal function in the obstructed kidney and also to evaluate the contralateral kidney. If residual renal function is adequate, pyeloplasty is the preferred treatment.

Contralateral renal anomalies can occur in 20%, including multicystic dysplastic kidney and renal agenesis. If the UPJ obstruction is severe in these cases, oligohydramnios will develop. Interestingly, unilateral UPJ obstruction may present with polyhydramnios. As opposed to a lower genitourinary tract obstruction, which has a 40% incidence of associated extrarenal anomalies, a UPJ obstruction has a lower incidence (12%) of gastrointestinal (esophageal and anal atresia, Hirschsprung's disease) complications, neural tube defects, and cardiovascular anomalies.

Notes

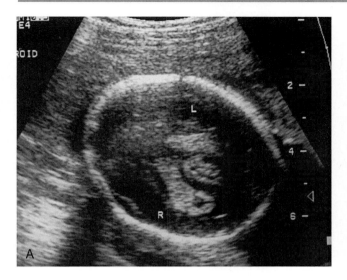

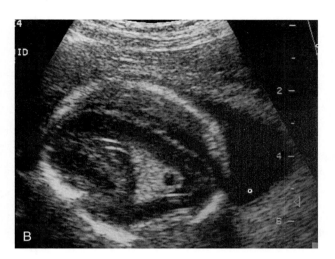

1. What is the finding in this second-trimester fetal head scan (Figs. A [axial] and B [sagittal]). What is the incidence of detection of this finding by ultrasound?

2. Can this be a normal finding? Is it associated with any karyotype abnormalities?

3. What factors are important when deciding whether amniocentesis is required?

4. Do any characteristics of these cysts (e.g., size and bilaterality) correlate with the presence of a karyotype abnormality?

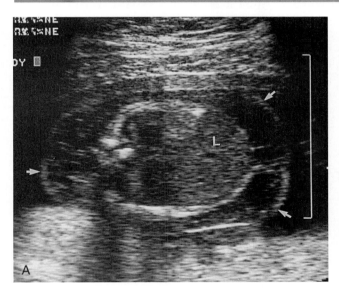

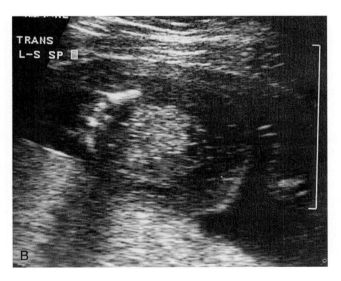

1. What is the chromosomal anomaly most likely to be present in this second-trimester fetus (Figs. A and B)? Figure A is an axial image of the upper body (L = liver). Figure B is an axial image of the pelvis.

2. What cardiovascular anomaly is associated?

3. Does the triple screen aid in the detection of this chromosomal anomaly?

4. Is this chromosomal anomaly associated with advanced maternal age?

CASE 5

Choroid Plexus Cysts

1. Choroid plexus cyst. The incidence is 0.2% to 2.5%.

2. Yes, often normal. Associated with trisomies 18 and 21.

3. Serum triple screen results, maternal age, and the presence of additional ultrasound findings.

4. No.

References

Gratton RJ, Hogge WA, Aston CE: Choroid plexus cysts and trisomy 18: Risk modification based on maternal age and multiple-marker screening. *Am J Obstet Gynecol* 175:1493–1497, 1996.

Reinsch RC: Choroid plexus cysts' association with trisomy: Prospective review of 16,059 patients. *Am J Obstet Gynecol* 176:1381–1383, 1997.

Cross-Reference
Ultrasound: THE REQUISITES, pp 221–224.

Comment

Choroid plexus cysts are detected in 0.2% to 2.5% of the population with prenatal ultrasonography and are often normal variants. Improvement in ultrasound technology has led to an increased ability to visualize these cysts; unfortunately, the management is controversial.

Choroid plexus cysts occur in fetuses with trisomy 18, but not in all cases. Furthermore, they also occur in 1% to 2% of the general population. Detection of a choroid plexus cyst requires a careful search for other findings of trisomy 18, including a strawberry-shaped skull, micrognathia, overlapping fingers, and clubfoot. Some studies report an increased incidence of trisomy 21. When another anomaly is detected on ultrasound, karyotype evaluation is recommended.

The controversy arises when isolated choroid plexus cysts are detected. Reports in the literature vary. One series reported that all fetuses with isolated choroid plexus cysts were normal at birth; other reports have revealed an increased incidence of karyotype abnormalities. Advanced maternal age, quoted as greater than or equal to 37 years, or an abnormal serum triple screen may dictate amniocentesis. However, the size of the cysts, the site (unilateral versus bilateral), the gestational age at detection, the gestational age at resolution, and the fetal sex cannot be used to predict the presence or absence of a karyotypic abnormality. Although most cysts resolve by 22 to 26 weeks of gestation, resolution does not reduce the likelihood of karyotypic abnormality.

Notes

CASE 6

Turner's Syndrome

1. Turner's syndrome.

2. Coarctation of the aorta.

3. Yes, but only 30% of cases will be detected.

4. No.

References

Saenger P: Turner's syndrome. *N Engl J Med* 335:1749–1754, 1996.

Shimizu T, Hashimoto K, Shimizu M, et al: Bilateral pleural effusion in the first trimester: A predictor of chromosomal anomaly and embryonic death? *Am J Obstet Gynecol* 177:470–471, 1997.

Wenstrom KD, Williamson RA, Grant SS: Detection of fetal Turner syndrome with multiple marker screening. *Am J Obstet Gynecol* 170:570–573, 1994.

Cross-Reference
Ultrasound: THE REQUISITES, pp 221; 232–233.

Comment

Turner's syndrome is the most common anomaly of sex chromosomes in females, with karyotype of 45,X0. The X chromosome is of maternal origin in two thirds of the cases and paternal origin in one third. Ninety-nine percent of all 45,X karyotype fetuses abort spontaneously. The chromosomal anomaly is *not* associated with advanced maternal age. The triple screen test may be abnormal. In most series, it is estimated that only 30% of cases will be detected.

Whereas many cases are discovered by amniocentesis or chorionic villus sampling, ultrasound findings can be helpful in detecting Turner's syndrome. Nuchal abnormalities range from nuchal thickening to full-blown cystic hygromas, with dilatation of the lymphatics arising from the posterior jugular sac. This case demonstrates a more diffuse lymphangiectasia (see Fig. A, denoted by arrows, and Fig. B). Cardiovascular malformations include coarctation of the aorta (<20%), often with a bicuspid aortic valve. Horseshoe kidney and other renal malformations are associated. The fetuses often have mild intrauterine growth retardation. A few cases of Turner's syndrome presenting in utero with transient pleural effusion have been described in the literature.

Almost 70% of cases of Turner's syndrome are lost from 16 weeks to term. Development of diffuse hydropic changes in the setting of a cystic hygroma is uniformly fatal. Survivors are monitored carefully for the multiple associated anomalies, which include hypothyroidism, otitis media, scoliosis, inflammatory bowel disease, mesenteric vascular anomalies, glucose intolerance, and hypertension. Estrogen is supplemented, beginning in the early teenage years. With assisted fertility, 50% to 60% of women with Turner's syndrome can become pregnant.

Notes

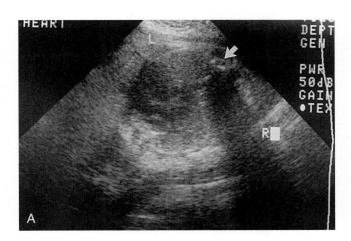

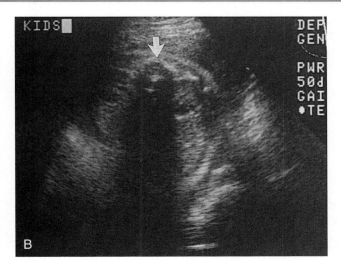

1. In this third-trimester fetus, what do you think is the most likely diagnosis for this lack of amniotic fluid and what is the most likely cause of death in the newborn? Figure A is an axial image of the fetal heart; Figure B is an axial image at the level of the kidneys (arrow = spine).

2. What factors predict the outcome in cases of spontaneous rupture of the membranes (SROM)?

3. What musculoskeletal complications result?

4. What is the potentially serious short-term complication of membrane rupture?

Oligohydramnios (Secondary to Spontaneous Rupture of the Membranes)

1. Severe oligohydramios secondary to SROM. Pulmonary hypoplasia.

2. Severity of fluid loss, gestational age at the time of rupture, and the length of exposure to oligohydramnios.

3. Limb deformities, including hip dysplasia and clubfoot.

4. Infection (chorioamnionitis).

References

Cunningham FG, MacDonald PC, Gant NF, et al: Placental disorders: Disease and abnormalities of the fetal membranes. In Cunningham FG, Williams JW (eds): *Williams Obstetrics,* 20th ed. Stamford, CT, Appleton & Lange, 1997, pp 664–665.

Kilbride HW, Yeast J, Thibeault DW: Obstetrics: Defining limits of survival: Lethal pulmonary hypoplasia after midtrimester premature rupture of membranes. *Am J Obstet Gynecol* 175:675–681, 1996.

Cross-Reference

Ultrasound: THE REQUISITES, pp 276–277.

Comment

This case of SROM shows that the degree of oligohydramnios can be severe (see Figs. A and B). The kidneys can frequently be seen (see Fig. B), and the urinary bladder can be identified. In cases of SROM, where the amniotic fluid index (AFI) is less than 1 cm, the duration of this severe exposure to oligohydramnios and the gestational age at the time of membrane rupture are predictors of fetal outcome. Fetal mortality is higher than 90% if membranes rupture before 25 weeks, and the exposure to severe oligohydramnios continues for more than 14 days. The mother is watched carefully for signs of infection (chorioamnionitis).

Twenty percent of cases of membrane rupture result in lethal pulmonary hypoplasia. In those fetuses that survive severe oligohydramnios due to membrane rupture, limb deformities can occur. In fact, 80% born after more than 2 weeks' exposure to severe oligohydramnios had such deformities, including clubfoot and congenital hip dysplasia.

In any case of newly diagnosed oligohydramnios with *intact* membranes, umbilical artery Doppler should be performed to exclude placental insufficiency. The systolic to diastolic ratio (S/D) is measured and compared with the normal range defined for each gestational age. In normal patients, the diastolic flow increases with increasing gestational age. In cases of intrauterine growth restriction, decreasing diastolic flow results in an *increase* in the S/D ratio. When the ratio falls above the 90th percentile, careful follow-up examinations are conducted to detect the absence or reversal of diastolic flow, which can prompt induction of delivery.

In gestations that extend beyond the expected due date, amniotic fluid can normally decrease. This may result occasionally in umbilical cord compression and fetal heart deceleration. Monitoring includes frequent AFI measurements and subjective quantitation of fluid volume, maternal assessment of fetal movement, and fetal non-stress cardiac testing.

Notes

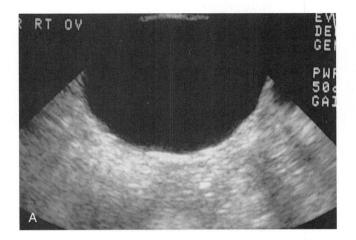

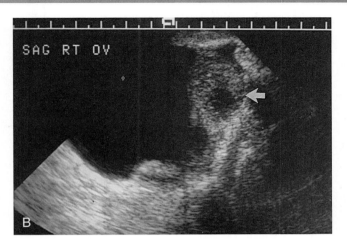

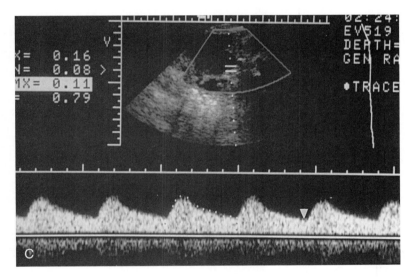

1. In this 50-year-old perimenopausal woman with a palpable right-sided pelvic mass, what is the most likely diagnosis and the differential diagnostic possibilities based on these ultrasound images of the right adnexa? (Figs. A and B: Arrow = the soft tissue component in Fig. B)

2. Does this spectral waveform from the soft tissue component raise concern regarding a malignancy (Fig. C)?

3. Does the impedance (i.e., resistive index [RI] and pulsatility index [PI]) aid in making the correct diagnosis?

4. Which benign ovarian masses may demonstrate high diastolic flow?

Ovarian Cancer (Cystadenocarcinoma)

1. Ovarian cancer (cystadenocarcinoma). The differential diagnoses are cystadenomas, tubo-ovarian abscess, endometriomas, corpus luteum cysts, and dermoids.

2. Yes, while occurring in some benign lesions, an arterial waveform with elevated diastolic flow (arrowhead) is seen in malignant ovarian lesions.

3. It can be helpful, but it is nonspecific.

4. Hormone-secreting or inflammatory lesions such as tubo-ovarian abscess, endometriomas, and dermoids.

References

Brown DL, Doubilet PM, Miller FH, et al: Benign and malignant ovarian masses: Selection of the most discriminating gray-scale and Doppler sonographic features. *Radiology* 208:103–110, 1998.

Hamper UM, Sheth S, Abbas FM, et al: Transvaginal color Doppler sonography of adnexal masses: Differences in blood flow impedance in benign and malignant lesions. *AJR Am J Roentgenol* 160:1225–1228, 1993.

Cross-Reference

Ultrasound: THE REQUISITES, pp 407–412.

Comment

Ultrasound is usually the first imaging modality for detection and characterization of ovarian cysts. Most simple cysts are benign follicles (usually <25 mm in long axis) that come and go with each menstrual cycle. Follow-up after one to two menstrual cycles is reasonable for any premenopausal woman with a simple or complex cyst, which could be a follicle or a hemorrhagic follicle to see if resolution occurs.

Ovarian cancer demonstrates a number of the ultrasound criteria for a malignant mass. The presence of a solid component or solid papillary mural projections (see Fig. B), particularly if they are *nonhyperechoic*, is worrisome. A hyperechoic solid component is seen more typically in a dermoid. If a fluid component is present, it is more commonly anechoic or hypoechoic. Septations may or may not be present in a malignant mass, but if present, they are usually 3 mm or thicker. The wall is often not discernible but can be thin or thick if seen. A malignant cyst is accompanied by ascites in 30% of cases and, when present, suggests spread to the pelvis (stage 2) or abdomen (stage 3 or 4).

Doppler ultrasound distinction of a benign from malignant ovarian mass has been shown to be nonpredictive. Doppler ultrasound was applied on the principle that low impedance flow should indicate a malignancy (see Fig. C). When arterial signals are detected, the systolic and diastolic components can be evaluated. Measurements include RI, also known as the Pourcelot index [(peak systolic velocity − end-diastolic velocity) ÷ peak systolic velocity] and PI [(peak systolic velocity − end-diastolic velocity) ÷ mean velocity]. The standard cutoff for malignancy is an RI less than 0.4 or a PI less than 1.0. It is not uncommon for a malignant lesion to have a borderline or low ratio that is suggestive of a malignancy. Conversely, arterial flow with systolic flow but little or no diastolic flow is a high resistance signal that is seen almost exclusively in benign lesions.

However, considerable overlap has been shown between benign and malignant mass when the spectral waveform shows an arterial waveform with a high diastolic component (low impedance). Benign masses that are endocrine-secreting or inflammatory may have this flow pattern, particularly tubo-ovarian abscesses, endometriomas, and ovarian dermoids.

Notes

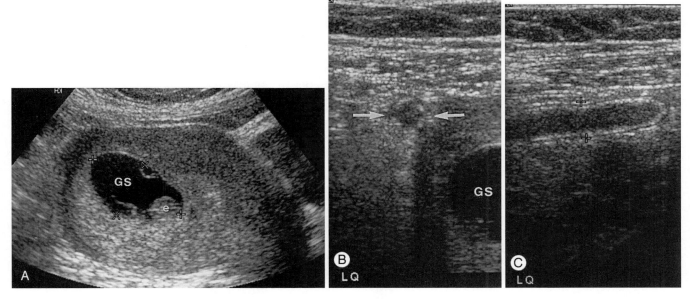

1. What is the most likely diagnosis in this transabdominal first trimester ultrasound examination (Figs. A to C)? Figure A is a sagittal midline image of the uterus. (GS = gestational sac; e = embryo with heart motion.) Figure B is an axial image of the upper uterine body. (GS = gestational sac; LQ = left quadrant; arrows = an adjacent extrauterine structure.) Figure C is a sagittal image to the right of the uterus, through the extrauterine structure in Figure B.

2. True or false: leukocytosis and right lower quadrant pain indicate appendicitis?

3. Does appendicitis have a higher mortality rate in pregnancy?

4. What are the complications of appendicitis in pregnancy?

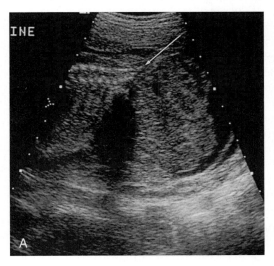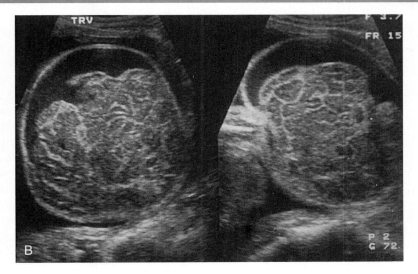

1. What is the abnormality shown on these sagittal (Fig. A) and axial (Fig. B) images of the fetal lower spine in this third-trimester fetus?

2. What factor increases the risk of malignancy?

3. What associated findings may be seen on prenatal ultrasound?

4. What are the hyperechoic foci that may be seen in this type of mass?

Appendicitis

1. Appendicitis.

2. False; leukocytosis can occur as part of a normal pregnancy.

3. Yes, particularly the third trimester.

4. Preterm delivery, spontaneous abortion, maternal-fetal sepsis, and even neonatal neurologic injury.

References
Coady DJ, Snyder JR, Subramanyam B: Appendiceal abscess in pregnancy: Diagnosis by ultrasound. *J Clin Ultrasound* 14:70–71, 1986.

Cunningham FG, MacDonald PC, Gant NF, et al: Medical and surgical complications in pregnancy. In Cunningham FG, Williams JW (eds): *Williams Obstetrics,* 20th ed. Stamford, CT, Appleton & Lange, 1997, pp 1151–1152.

Hansen GC, Toot PJ, Lynch CO: Subtle ultrasound signs of appendicitis in a pregnant patient: A case report. *J Reprod Med* 38:223–224, 1993.

Cross-Reference
Ultrasound: THE REQUISITES, pp 457–458.

Comment
Appendicitis occurs in 1 in 1500 pregnant women. It can develop in the first, second, or third trimester. Unfortunately, the symptoms of appendicitis are also symptoms that occur in a normal pregnancy. Leukocytosis and nausea are common. The enlarging uterus can cause severe right lower quadrant pain owing to round ligament strain. The clinical differential diagnosis of right lower quadrant pain in pregnancy includes appendicitis, renal calculus, pyelonephritis, placental abruption, degeneration of myoma, ovarian cyst, and torsion.

Ultrasound has been used to make the diagnosis, avoiding the ionizing radiation of computed tomography. Early in pregnancy, the inflamed appendix may be visualized as a noncompressible tubular structure measuring 6 mm or greater, as shown in this case (see Figs. B and C, +'s denote the diameter of 10 mm in Fig. C). Pain often occurs directly over this area. In the setting of perforation, a collection of peritoneal fluid may be detected. As the uterus enlarges, the appendix can move superiorly and toward the flanks.

If the diagnosis is highly suspected, surgery is advised. In one series, 50% of those who underwent surgery had appendicitis. If the diagnosis is missed, peritonitis results. In the third trimester, this has a poor prognosis, and maternal mortality is approximately 5%. Other complications include preterm labor, spontaneous abortion, and even fetal neurologic injury if maternal-fetal sepsis results.

Notes

Sacrococcygeal Teratoma

1. Sacrococcygeal teratoma.

2. Diagnosis after 2 to 4 months of *neonatal* age.

3. Bladder displacement, hydronephrosis, and polyhydramnios.

4. Calcifications.

Reference
Sheth S, Nussbaum SR, Sanders RC, et al: Prenatal diagnosis of sacrococcygeal teratoma: Sonographic-pathologic correlation. *Radiology* 169:131-136, 1988.

Cross-Reference
Ultrasound: THE REQUISITES, p 233.

Comment
Sacrococcygeal teratoma is the most common congenital tumor in the newborn. Women often present with a large-for-dates uterus owing to polyhydramnios. The diagnosis is important, because most pregnancies result in premature delivery. More important, if the mass is not diagnosed, vaginal delivery may lead to dystocia and intratumoral hemorrhage owing to a traumatic delivery. Cesarean section is often necessary.

The mass may be one of four subtypes: (1) exterior with a minimal presacral component, (2) exterior with a significant presacral component, (3) both exterior and presacral, and (4) predominantly presacral. The latter has the worst prognosis and may not be detected at birth; the risk of malignancy increases with age after delivery (particularly after 2 to 4 months of age).

On ultrasound, a mass that is usually cystic and solid is seen in the region of the fetal sacrum. Calcifications are often present, owing to fragments of bone or dystrophic calcification. A review of several cases demonstrated three ultrasound patterns: (1) predominantly solid with small anechoic areas (as shown here), (2) a unilocular cystic mass, or (3) a mixed solid and cystic mass. Although the presacral component may be visualized on ultrasound, the internal component can go undetected, even when it is large. There is little or no distortion of the sacral spine (see Fig. A) but the tumor may spread into the spinal canal. Associated findings are important; if they include bladder displacement and hydronephrosis, severe renal dysfunction with oligohydramnios may result. Furthermore, because these tumors may be very vascular (often appreciated with Doppler ultrasound), the following can develop: high-output problems for the fetus, massive polyhydramnios necessitating therapeutic amniocentesis, placentomegaly, and hydrops.

Notes

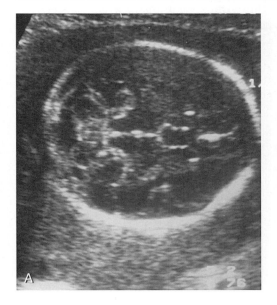

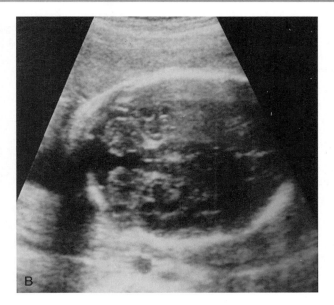

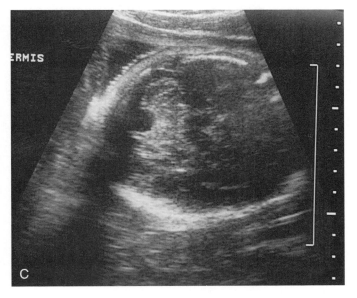

1. Three mid–second-trimester fetal brains with axial scans of the posterior fossae (Figs. A to C). Which are abnormal, and what are their diagnoses?

2. Does the presence of ventriculomegaly with this disorder have any prognostic significance?

3. Which portion of the cerebellar vermis fuses last?

4. When is the cerebellar vermis completely fused?

Dandy-Walker Malformation

1. A is normal; B is complete; and C has partial absence of the cerebellar vermis in Dandy-Walker malformation.

2. Yes, there is an inverse relationship between the presence of hydrocephalus and chromosomal anomalies.

3. Fusion begins superiorly and continues inferiorly.

4. Embryologically the vermis may fuse by the end of the 15th week. Using ultrasound, an open vermis may be seen in normal patients before 18 weeks.

References

Baumeister LA, Hertzberg BS, McNally PJ, et al: Fetal fourth ventricle: US appearance and frequency of depiction. *Radiology* 192:333–336, 1994.

Bromley B, Nadel AS, Paulker S, et al: Closure of the cerebellar vermis: Evaluation with second trimester US. *Radiology* 193:761–763, 1994.

Chang MC, Russell SA, Callen PW, et al: Sonographic detection of inferior vermian agenesis in Dandy-Walker malformations: Prognostic implications. *Radiology* 192:765–770, 1994.

Cross-Reference

Ultrasound: THE REQUISITES, pp 220–221.

Comment

Dandy-Walker malformation consists of variable degrees of cerebellar vermian agenesis (see Figs. B and C), dilatation of the fourth ventricle, and enlargement of the posterior fossa. The cisterna magna communicates with the fourth ventricle. Ventriculomegaly may be present and was reported in 24% to 71% of cases. Nyberg described an inverse relationship between the presence of chromosomal anomalies and ventriculomegaly.

The cerebellar vermis is open early in gestation and closes in most normal patients by 18 weeks of age. Accordingly, an open cerebellar vermis on prenatal ultrasound *cannot* be considered abnormal until 18 weeks' gestation. Ultrasound criteria for a normal posterior fossa include a cisterna magna from 2 to 10 mm and a bilobed cerebellum. The normal fourth ventricle can be seen 70% of the time in the mid-second trimester and measures 3.5 × 3.9 mm on average. The posterior fossa should be imaged in an axial plane; semicoronal imaging toward the cervical spine often yields spurious enlargement of the cisterna magna.

Because approximately 75% of afflicted fetuses with Dandy-Walker malformation have concomitant anomalies, the mortality rate has been reported to be as high as 70%. Chromosomal anomalies are present in almost one third of cases, including trisomy 13, 18, and 21.

Additional central nervous system abnormalities include agenesis of the corpus callosum, aqueductal stenosis, microcephaly, and encephalocele. Cardiac, genitourinary, and facial malformations as well as polydactyly are common.

Notes

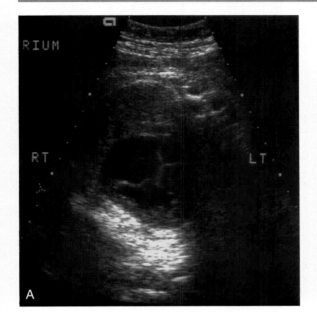

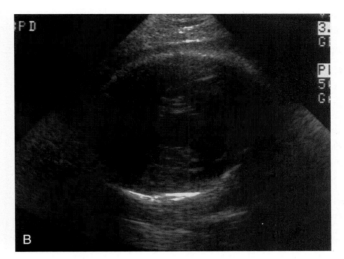

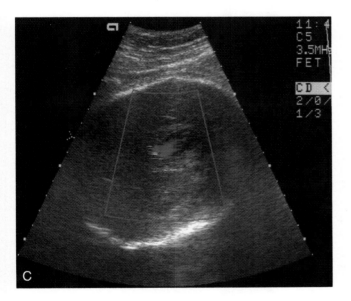

1. How does Figure A of the fetal heart relate to Figures B and C of the fetal head?

2. What are the central nervous system (CNS) complications?

3. Are other cardiovascular malformations associated with this cerebral abnormality?

4. When does this malformation present in utero?

Central Nervous System Arteriovenous Malformation

1. Cardiomegaly resulting from high-output heart failure due to an intracranial arteriovenous malformation (AVM).

2. Cerebral anoxia, porencephaly, and hydrocephalus.

3. Yes, coarctation of the aorta and transposition of the great vessels.

4. Usually after 30 weeks.

Reference

Comstock CH, Kirk JS: Arteriovenous malformations: Locations and evolution in the fetal brain. *J Ultrasound Med* 10:361–365, 1991.

Cross-Reference

Ultrasound: THE REQUISITES, p 225.

Comment

Intracranial fetal AVMs almost always involve the vein of Galen, as shown in this case. Although traditionally called an "aneurysm," this malformation represents a direct arteriovenous anastomosis or arteriovenous fistula. Anterior and posterior circulation supply the malformation, stealing blood from the cerebral vasculature; the vein of Galen drains the malformation and dilates. The outcome is usually poor, particularly if high-output heart failure develops, as shown by cardiomegaly in Figure A; the heart is greater than one half of the diameter of the chest. Associated cardiovascular malformations include coarctation of the aorta and transposition of the great vessels.

On prenatal ultrasound, these malformations do not become apparent until the third trimester, usually after 30 weeks. A cystic structure is identified posterior to the foramen of Monro (superior to the third ventricle), just superior and posterior to the thalamus (see Fig. B). The structure is generally larger than 2.5 cm in its shortest diameter and fills with color Doppler (see Fig. C). Arterial or high venous flow is detected with spectral Doppler, depending on the site of interrogation. Dilated intracerebral vessels may be detected around the AVM. The head circumference is normal. Hydrocephalus, usually seen in the neonate with a vein of Galen AVM, is not always present prenatally.

Because of the high flow through the AVM or possibly owing to pressure necrosis, cerebral anoxia may lead to microinfarcts and periventricular leukomalacia. The fetal heart or right ventricle is usually enlarged. Hydrops fetalis results from high-output heart failure and can cause pulmonary hypoplasia from pleural effusions. The prognosis relates to the presence of heart failure rather than to the size of the lesion.

Notes

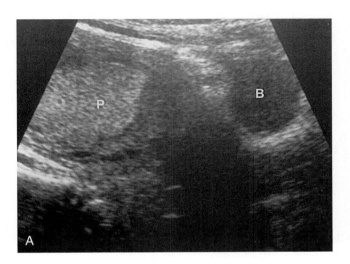

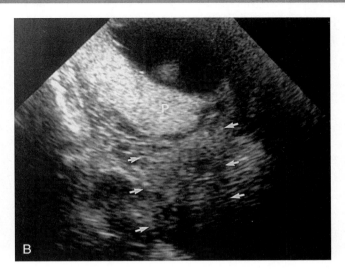

1. In this late second-trimester pregnancy, Figures A and B are transabdominal images of the lower uterine segment (LUS). Which is more diagnostic and why? P = placenta.

2. What are the best imaging techniques to evaluate for a placenta previa?

3. Can the diagnosis of placenta previa be made via a transabdominal scan?

4. Name three complications of placenta previa.

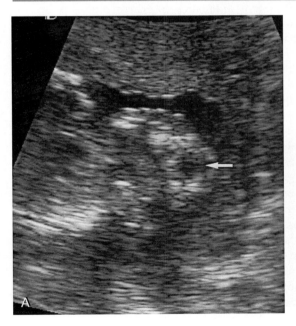

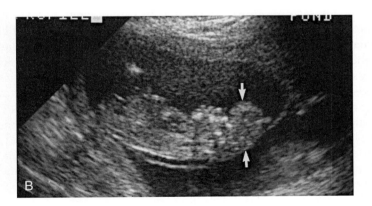

1. What is the diagnosis in these two early second-trimester pregnancies: Figure A (fetus A) is of the fetal head in sagittal projection and Figure B (fetus B, one of twins) a sagittal image of the entire fetus? What structures are labeled by arrows in the fetal heads of Figures A and B?

2. When can this disorder be reliably detected by ultrasound?

3. When does the neural tube close?

4. Which dietary deficiency is associated with this disorder?

Placenta Previa

1. Figure B. The urinary bladder is empty.

2. Translabial and transvaginal ultrasound with an empty bladder.

3. Yes, if the bladder is empty.

4. Hemorrhage, placental invasion (accreta), and intrauterine growth restriction.

References

Hertzberg BS, Bowie JD, Carroll BA, et al: Diagnosis of placenta previa during the third trimester: Role of transperineal sonography. *AJR Am J Roentgenol* 159:83–87, 1992.

Mabie WC: Placenta Previa. *Clin Perinatol* 19:425–435, 1992.

Cross-Reference

Ultrasound: THE REQUISITES, pp 323–327; 329; 339.

Comment

Implantation of the placenta over the cervix (Fig. B—*arrows*) is described as placenta previa. Placenta previa can be complete (the internal os is covered by placenta), partial (partial coverage of the os), or marginal (the placental edge is at the margin of the os). A low-lying placenta (within 2 cm of the internal os) does not reach the internal os but may be clinically important because it can be incorporated into the dilated cervix at the time of delivery, leading to hemorrhage.

Complications can occur in addition to hemorrhage. An anterior placenta may invade the uterine wall—(placenta accreta), particularly in patients with a previa and a history of cesarean section. Fetal complications include intrauterine growth restriction and subsequent development of cerebral palsy. Even the low-lying placenta may increase the incidence of small for gestational age fetuses.

Many cases can be diagnosed with transabdominal ultrasound. The bladder must be empty to make an accurate diagnosis. A distended bladder or uterine contraction can cause a false-positive result by compressing the LUS and making a low-lying placenta appear like a placenta previa. Translabial and transvaginal imaging after bladder emptying are often necessary to adequately visualize the LUS, particularly in the third trimester. The transvaginal probe should be inserted only partially in order to avoid direct contact with the cervix.

Most cases diagnosed early in pregnancy resolve, probably because of placental remodeling owing to poor blood supply of the LUS. Follow-up imaging is required in the third trimester (~30 weeks). A cesarean section is performed for a persistent placenta previa.

Notes

Anencephaly

1. Anencephaly. A: orbit; B: angiomatous stroma.

2. May be seen as early as 8 weeks but is seen reliably by the second trimester.

3. 24 days of fetal life; 38 menstrual days.

4. Folic acid.

Reference

Goldstein RB, Filly RA: Prenatal diagnosis of anencephaly: Spectrum of sonographic appearances and distinction from the amniotic band syndrome. *AJR Am J Roentgenol* 151:547–550, 1988.

Cross-Reference

Ultrasound: THE REQUISITES, pp 207–209.

Comment

With an overall frequency of 1 in 1000, anencephaly is one of the most common neural tube defects. The incidence varies in different parts of the world. The cerebral cortex and skull are absent; orbits, brainstem, and skull base are present. In some cases, "angiomatous stroma" or vascular, dysmorphic tissue may cover the brainstem, as shown in Figure B. Like other central nervous system anomalies, polyhydramnios is associated, particularly later in the gestation. The disorder is incompatible with life.

A deficiency of maternal folic acid has been shown to increase the risk of neural tube defects. It is recommended that women begin folic acid supplementation before becoming pregnant to decrease the risk of anencephaly and other neural tube defects.

Ultrasound demonstrates the absence of a calvarium and brain above the orbits (see Fig. A), cephalad to the brainstem. Whereas this may be detected as early as 8 weeks, it is diagnosed more reliably in the early second trimester.

Routine screening of maternal serum α-fetoprotein (AFP) is performed between 15 and 20 weeks as part of the serum triple screen (AFP, estriol, and human chorionic gonadotropin). The serum AFP is usually elevated in anencephaly, using either 2.0 or 2.5 multiples of the median (MOM) as the cutoff for detection. It is important that the pregnancy is dated accurately, as the levels vary with gestational age. The serum AFP level will also be abnormal in multiple gestations and obese women. The differential diagnosis for an elevated maternal AFP in pregnancy includes other open defects, such as gastroschisis, as well as fetal-maternal hemorrhage, maternal hepatitis, or maternal hepatocellular carcinoma.

Notes

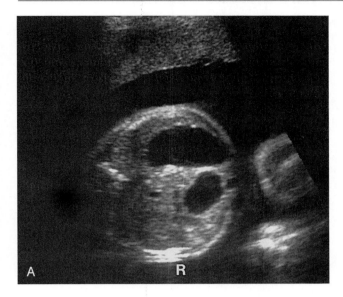

1. What are the two cystic structures shown on this axial image of the upper abdomen in this 24-week-old fetus (Fig. A; R = right side of the fetus)?

2. What is the most common cause of this finding?

3. What chromosomal anomaly is associated?

4. What prenatal complications are associated?

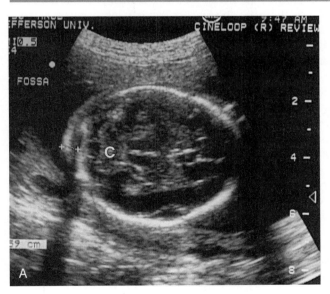

1. What is being measured posterior to the occiput in this 18-week-old fetus (Fig. A, +'s)? It measures slightly less than 6 mm. Is this normal?

2. What are the proposed etiologies of thickening in this region?

3. What is the significance of thickening of this region that resolves later in the gestation?

4. In fetuses with an abnormal thickness and normal karyotype, is there any other significance?

Duodenal Atresia

1. Stomach (larger) and duodenal bulb (smaller).

2. Duodenal atresia.

3. Down syndrome.

4. Polyhydramnios (30%) and premature birth (45%).

Reference

Grosfeld JL, Rescorla RJ: Duodenal atresia and stenosis: Reassessment of treatment and outcome based on antenatal diagnosis, pathologic variance and long-term follow-up. *World J Surg* 17:301–309, 1993.

Cross-Reference

Ultrasound: THE REQUISITES, pp 258–259.

Comment

Pathologically, a duodenal obstruction can be intrinsic or extrinsic. Extrinsic causes include annular pancreas, preduodenal portal vein, Ladd's bands, and malrotation. Duodenal obstruction is most commonly caused by duodenal atresia or stenosis, which is classically associated with Down syndrome (trisomy 21). However, only 30% of the fetuses with duodenal atresia or stenosis have trisomy 21. Intrinsic stenosis/atresia is further categorized as mucosal atresia (type I), fibrous cord (type II), or complete separation of the duodenum (type III) usually near the ampulla of Vater. Concomitant biliary duct anomalies occur most commonly in the type III subset.

Prenatal ultrasound of a duodenal obstruction demonstrates a "double bubble," corresponding to a dilated stomach and duodenal bulb, as shown here. Polyhydramnios develops in 30% of cases (see Fig. A), and 45% are born premature. Both the "double bubble" and polyhydramnios are often not detected until after 24 weeks. This is surprising, because the duodenal obstruction is typically complete. Perhaps it is related to the examiner's failure to appreciate the second bubble, if small, as a distended duodenum and the slow accumulation of amniotic fluid, which may not truly increase until later in the pregnancy.

At least 50% of all fetuses with atresia or stenosis may have an additional anomaly, most commonly a complex cardiac malformation. The cardiac defects cause most of the deaths in these children, thus although prenatal detection may lead to earlier gastrointestinal surgery, the outcome may still be poor. Other anomalies include esophageal atresia, imperforate anus, renal malformations, and biliary atresia. Once duodenal atresia is detected, a careful search should be conducted for other anomalies with prenatal ultrasound, including a fetal echocardiogram.

Notes

Nuchal Skin Measurement—Second Trimester

1. Nuchal thickness. Yes.

2. Lymphatic obstruction and cardiac disease.

3. Still carries increased risk of chromosomal anomaly.

4. Yes, cardiac malformations, various syndromes, and other complications are associated.

References

Landwehr JB, Johnson MP, Hume RF, et al: Abnormal nuchal findings on screening ultrasonography: Aneuploidy stratification on the basis of ultrasonographic anomaly and gestational age at detection. *Am J Obstet Gynecol* 175:995–999, 1996.

Reynderes CS, Pauker SP, Benacerraf BR: First trimester isolated fetal nuchal lucency: Significance and outcome. *J Ultrasound Med* 16:101–105, 1997.

Cross-Reference

Ultrasound: THE REQUISITES, pp 221–222; 234.

Comment

Nuchal thickening is a marker for chromosomal anomalies. In the second trimester (16 to 22 weeks), the nuchal thickness should be no greater than 6 mm. This measurement is performed in the axial plane at the level of the thalami. The transducer is *slightly* tilted so that the frontal region is more cephalad, and the posterior fossa is imaged. The region from the surface of the skin to the surface of the occipital skull is measured.

The etiology of nuchal thickening is controversial. Some believe that it is caused by edema owing to cardiovascular abnormalities. In fact, increased nuchal translucency in the first trimester has been shown to be more prevalent in fetuses with major cardiac defects. Lymphatic obstruction is another proposed etiology.

Nuchal thickening and cystic hygromas can resolve as the gestation evolves; although, this does not decrease the risk of a karyotype abnormality or change the prognosis.

Nuchal thickening and translucencies can be seen in embryos/fetuses with no chromosomal anomalies. However, those with normal karyotypes have a higher risk of other malformations and syndromes, including Noonan's syndrome, Joubert's syndrome, and multiple pterygium syndrome. In addition, there is an increased risk of spontaneous miscarriage and premature delivery.

Notes

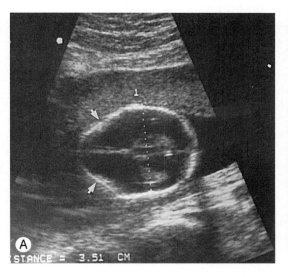

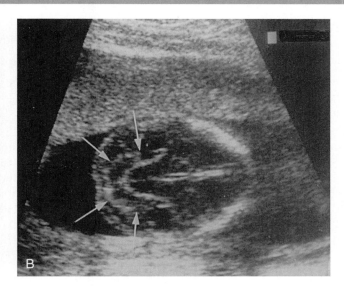

1. Which is the most likely cause of the fetal head anomalies in these two second-trimester fetuses (Figs. A and B are axial images)?

2. Which of the head anomalies in this disorder are more common before 24 weeks? After 24 weeks?

3. When does the distal spine ossify in normal fetuses?

4. Name two associated musculoskeletal findings.

C A S E   1 8

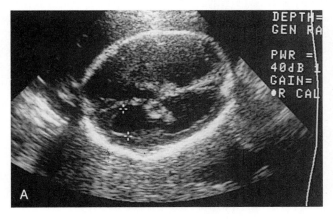

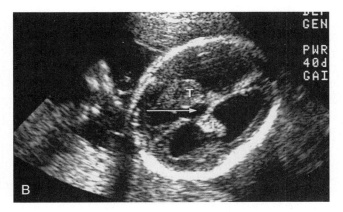

1. In this second-trimester fetus, what is the most likely etiology for its hydrocephalus (Fig. A, +'s measuring one of the dilated lateral ventricles)?

2. What percentage of causes of fetal hydrocephalus does this comprise?

3. Are other anomalies associated, and are they significant?

4. Is the outcome generally good?

Myelomeningocele

1. Open spina bifida (meningocele and myelomeningocele).

2. Before 24 weeks: lemon head sign and banana-shaped cerebellum. After 24 weeks: ventriculomegaly and obliterated cisterna magna.

3. After 22 weeks.

4. Clubfoot and scoliosis/kyphosis.

References

Babcook CJ, Drake CM, Goldstein RB: Spinal level of fetal myelomeningocele: Does it influence ventricular size? *AJR Am J Roentgenol* 169:207–210, 1997.

Babcook CJ, Goldstein RB, Barth RA, et al: Prevalence of ventriculomegaly in association with myelomeningocele: Correlation with gestational age and severity of posterior fossa deformity. *Radiology* 190:703–707, 1994.

Budorick NE, Pretorius DH, Nelson TR: Sonography of the fetal spine: Technique, imaging findings and clinical implications. *AJR Am J Roentgenol* 164:421–428, 1995.

Cross-Reference

Ultrasound: THE REQUISITES, pp 225–232.

Comment

Meningocele and myelomeningocele comprise the spectrum of open spina bifida; the latter contains nerve fibers in addition to meninges and cerebrospinal fluid. These spine abnormalities can occur anywhere, but they are much more common in the lumbosacral region. Almost all are associated with a posterior fossa deformity (Chiari II-hindbrain malformation).

Four cranial abnormalities are associated. As a result of the posterior fossa deformity (see Fig. B), the cerebellum becomes banana shaped (usually seen before 24 weeks), and the cisterna magna effaced (more common after 24 weeks). Before 24 weeks, the cranium may have a lemon shape (see Fig. A) (concave frontal bones). Ventriculomegaly is present in 70% to 80% of fetuses and 90% of infants with this disorder and becomes more prevalent after 24 weeks' gestation. It probably results from an obstruction of cerebrospinal flow by the posterior fossa deformity as the presence of ventriculomegaly correlates with the severity of the posterior fossa defect. However, unlike infants in whom the degree of postoperative ventricular dilatation correlates with the level of the neural tube defect, the level in the fetus does not correlate with ventricular size.

Notes

Aqueductal Stenosis

1. Aqueductal stenosis.

2. 20%.

3. Yes; yes.

4. No, mortality is 40%. Only 10% of these children will be physically and neuropsychologically normal.

Reference

Levitsky DB, Mack LA, Nyberg DA, et al: Fetal aqueductal stenosis diagnosed sonographically: How grave is the prognosis? *AJR Am J Roentgenol* 164:725–730, 1995.

Cross-Reference

Ultrasound: THE REQUISITES, pp 211–214.

Comment

Aqueductal stenosis is the cause of 20% of the cases of in utero hydrocephalus. It can be congenital, either X-linked or a part of an autosomal recessive disorder. Additionally, in utero infection and hemorrhage can result in aqueductal stenosis. This is a diagnosis of exclusion, once other causes of hydrocephalus have been investigated and ruled out.

The ultrasound findings, as shown by this case, are enlargement of the lateral and third ventricles (Fig. B: arrow = third ventricle; T = thalami). The third ventricle can usually be identified in the third trimester and sometimes in the second trimester. It is normally less than or equal to 2 mm in diameter and is situated between the thalami. In aqueductal stenosis, the dilatation is usually marked, ranging from 3 to 25 mm (mean, 10 mm). Measurement of the atria of the lateral ventricles ranges from 15 to 70 mm. Thinning of the fronto-parietal cortex may correlate with the degree of developmental impairment.

Associated anomalies can occur in 30% of cases, warranting a careful search with prenatal ultrasound. These anomalies include tracheoesophageal fistula, cleft palate, cardiac malformations (ventricular septal defect, atrial septal defect, transposition of the great vessels), renal agenesis, vertebral abnormalities, and polydactyly. In addition, adduction of the thumb, positioned on the palmar surface, is a characteristic hand configuration associated with aqueductal stenosis. Macrocephaly may dictate the requirement for cesarean section delivery.

Shunting is usually performed postnatally. The mortality rate is nevertheless high at 40%, owing to the associated anomalies; deaths occur in utero, in the neonatal period, and later. Most of the surviving children have degrees of developmental impairment, which relate to the central nervous system malformations.

Notes

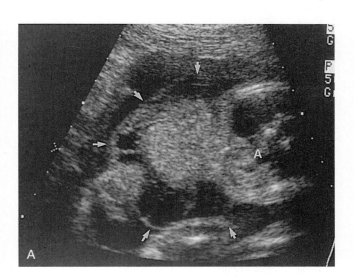

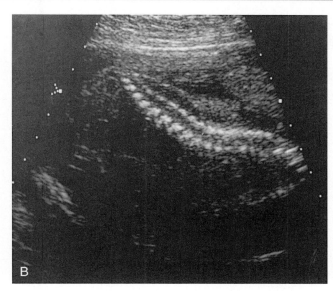

1. In this second-trimester fetus, what is the most likely diagnosis and the differential diagnoses of the abnormality (arrows) projecting anteriorly from the abdomen (A) (Fig. A)?

2. Which entity has associated chromosomal anomalies?

3. How does the cord insertion aid in distinguishing the etiology?

4. At what gestational age can an omphalocele be reliably diagnosed?

Omphalocele

1. Omphalocele. The differential diagnoses are gastroschisis and limb-body wall complex.

2. Omphalocele.

3. In small omphaloceles, usually containing only bowel, the cord inserts centrally. In large omphaloceles and in the limb-body wall complex, the cord insertion is displaced to the side of the defect. In gastroschisis, the normal cord insertion is identified away from the defect.

4. Because of normal midgut herniation in the first trimester, the diagnosis of omphalocele must await the second trimester.

Reference

Emanuel PG, Garcia GI, Angtuaco TL: Prenatal detection of anterior abdominal wall defects with ultrasound. *Radiographics* 15:517–530, 1995.

Cross-Reference

Ultrasound: THE REQUISITES, pp 265–267.

Comment

An omphalocele is a midline anterior abdominal wall defect that may contain varying amounts of abdominal contents. In those containing only bowel, the primitive body stalk or normal midgut herniation persisted beyond 12 weeks. If the liver or other organs herniate into the omphalocele, the lateral body wall failed to migrate, thus precluding closure. A diagnosis with prenatal ultrasound is possible only after 12 weeks, when the normal herniation of the midgut has resolved.

In contradistinction to gastroschisis and the limb-body wall complex, the umbilical cord inserts into the apex of the defect in a small omphalocele. With larger omphaloceles, the cord insertion can be identified at the edge of the omphalocele. A covering membrane of peritoneum is present. In the larger defects, such as that shown in Figure A, the hyperechoic areas can be either non–fluid-filled bowel or organs such as the liver. Cystic structures may be either fluid-filled bowel or ascites. This case demonstrates an additional scoliosis of the thoracolumbar spine (Fig. B). Unlike most limb-body wall defects where the scoliosis is often associated with a spinal defect, the scoliosis in large omphaloceles (when present) represents an otherwise normal spine that "collapses" because of a lack of abdominal contents.

Associated malformations are present in up to 90% of cases. Chromosomal anomalies are present in 30% to 40% of cases (most commonly trisomy 13 or 18), particularly those with small bowel involvement. Syndromes that include omphaloceles are Beckwith-Wiede-mann syndrome, bladder exstrophy, and pentalogy of Cantrell. Central nervous system, cardiac, gastrointestinal, and genitourinary malformations may be associated. Malrotation and intestinal atresia, atrial septal defect, ventriculoseptal defect, tetralogy of Fallot, and ectopia cordis are among the specific anomalies reported. The presence of a concurrent malformation, particularly chromosomal or cardiac, increases mortality to almost 100%.

Notes

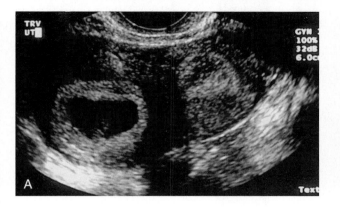

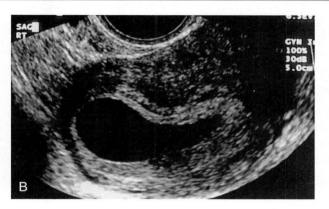

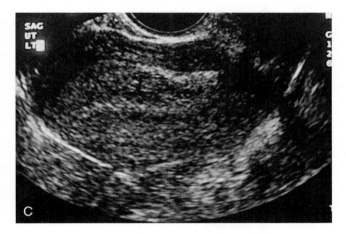

1. This is a first-trimester transabdominal ultrasound study (Figs. A to C). Figure A is an axial image of the uterus. Figure B is a sagittal image of the uterus toward the right, and Figure C is a sagittal image of the uterus toward the left. What is your diagnosis?

2. Which uterine anomaly has the highest incidence of reproductive dysfunction? *Septum*

3. Which uterine anomalies are most commonly associated with *early* pregnancy loss? With second- or third-trimester pregnancy loss?

4. Which uterine anomaly has an increased risk of cervical and vaginal neoplasia?

Congenital Uterine Anomalies and Pregnancy

1. Bicornuate or septate uterus with a pregnancy in the right horn.

2. Septate uterus.

3. Early loss: septate and bicornuate uteri, diethylstilbestrol (DES)-related anomalies, and unicornuate with a rudimentary horn. Later loss: bicornuate uterus.

4. DES-related anomalies.

Reference

Wagner BJ, Woodward PJ: Magnetic resonance evaluation of congenital uterine anomalies. *Semin Ultrasound CT MR* 15:4–17, 1994.

Cross-Reference

Ultrasound: THE REQUISITES, pp 364, 385.

Comment

A large study of fertile and infertile women showed that the most common uterine anomalies are bicornuate (39%) and septate (34%) uteri. Didelphic comprised 11%, arcuate 7%, unicornuate 5% and hypoplastic 4%. All have a higher incidence of renal anomalies, including unilateral agenesis and ptosis.

Uterine anomalies are present in a higher frequency in infertile women. Depending on the congenital anomaly, women may have difficulty with conception, early pregnancy loss, or later complications such as intrauterine growth restriction (IUGR). The septate uterus has the highest incidence of reproductive difficulties (67%).

Problems with conception may occur with a septate uterus. This may be caused by implantation on the septum, which has a decreased blood supply, particularly the inferior fibrous portion. Early pregnancy loss also occurs; other anomalies that have an increased incidence of early pregnancy loss include a unicornuate uterus with a rudimentary horn and DES-related anomalies.

This case shows an early intrauterine gestation within the right horn of a bicornuate uterus (see Figs. A to C). Pregnancy loss occurs more frequently with a bicornuate uterus than with a uterine didelphys or a unicornuate uterus. The loss can occur in the first 20 weeks or later in the second or third trimester.

Women whose mothers used DES during pregnancy can have a T-shaped uterus or uterine cavity constrictions that are not amenable to surgical correction. In addition, they have an increased risk of cervical and vaginal malignancies. There are no associated genitourinary anomalies in the DES-related uterine malformations.

Notes

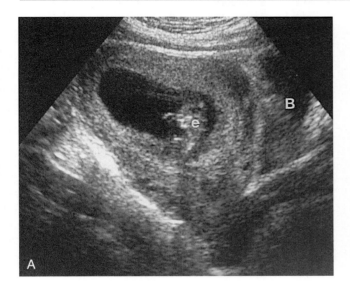

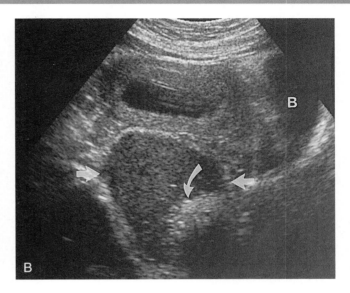

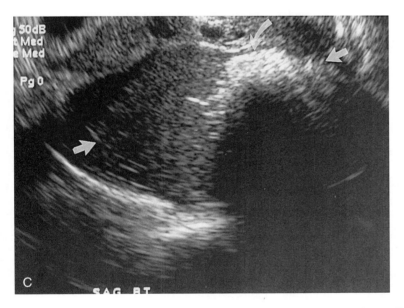

1. In this first-trimester ultrasound examination (Figs. A to C), where is the abnormality (denoted by arrows) and what is the most likely diagnosis? Figure A is a transabdominal sagittal midline scan showing a living embryo (e) within an intrauterine gestational sac (B = urinary bladder). Figure B is a transabdominal sagittal scan to the right of midline showing a portion of the intrauterine gestational sac and an area denoted by arrows (curved arrow = a portion of the abnormality; B = urinary bladder). Figure C is a transvaginal study to the right, denoting the abnormality in Figure B (arrows and curved arrow).

2. In a first-trimester pregnancy, what are the most likely differential diagnoses of a mass detected lateral to the uterus?

3. Do extrauterine masses need to be removed during pregnancy?

4. If necessary to perform surgery to remove an extrauterine mass, what would be the best time for this operation?

Normal First-Trimester Intrauterine Pregnancy with Extrauterine Mass, a Cystic Teratoma (Dermoid)

1. An extrauterine mass, probably a cystic teratoma (dermoid).

2. If cystic, a prominent corpus luteum cyst or nonfunctioning ovarian cyst. If complex, predominantly cystic, a hemorrhagic cyst, endometrioma, cystic teratoma, neoplasm, either benign or malignant or rarely a concomitant ectopic pregnancy. If solid, a solid ovarian mass (benign or malignant), exophytic fibroid, ovarian torsion, or pelvic kidney.

3. If large, yes.

4. In the early to mid-second trimester, after the fourth month of pregnancy.

Reference

Eastman NJ, Helman LM (eds): *Williams Obstetrics*, 13th ed. Stanford, CT, Appleton Century Crofts 1966, pp 909–919.

Cross-Reference

Ultrasound: THE REQUISITES, pp 396–402.

Comment

Extrauterine masses associated with pregnancy can be detected by both transabdominal and transvaginal ultrasound examinations. Their detection is commonly an incidental finding, although occasionally the physical examination may suggest the abnormality. These masses are usually ovarian in origin. When cystic, they may be a corpus luteum cyst or nonfunctioning ovarian cyst. If complex, they can be a hemorrhagic cyst, cystic teratoma, or neoplasm (cystadenomas and cystadenocarcinomas). Although endometriomas are often associated with infertility, they may be seen following pregnancy and can be extraovarian or, less commonly, ovarian. Solid masses are often exophytic fibroids, solid benign ovarian masses, ovarian carcinoma, or a pelvic kidney. Abscesses can vary in their appearance and typically present with significant symptomatology. A hydrosalpinx appears tubular, especially on a transvaginal study. Ovarian torsion is more often solid and related to pain. Although usually associated with a lead mass, necrosis tends to produce an amorphous solid appearance.

This case shows a fairly typical appearance for one of the more common extrauterine masses (a cystic teratoma [dermoid]) detected during pregnancy (see Figs. B and C). The mass is well circumscribed and has low-level internal echoes with a hyperechoic area with shadowing distally denoting a "dermoid plug" (curved arrow).

Ovarian tumors may cause complications during pregnancy. These tumors are associated with the increased possibility of a spontaneous abortion; they may undergo torsion; and they may pose obstacles to vaginal delivery. Even after spontaneous labor, the tumors may cause disturbances in the postpartum period. Although all types of ovarian tumors may complicate pregnancy and delivery, most of them are cystic. They occur once in every 81 pregnancies, but the ones that are of sufficient size to constitute a hazard to pregnancy are considered with an incidence of only 1 in 328. Dermoids have been described comparatively frequently. The most frequent and serious complication of ovarian cystic masses is torsion, which frequently occurs after 9 weeks. The cysts may rupture and extrude their contents into the peritoneal cavity during spontaneous labor or as a result of operative interference. If the tumor blocks the pelvis, it can rupture the uterus or be forced into the vagina and occasionally even into the rectum.

Many ovarian tumors complicating pregnancy are unsuspected. Ultrasound can detect extrauterine tumors, particularly smaller ones that may not cause many of these complications. However, if these tumors are clinically considered to be large enough to cause problems (usually >4 to 5 cm), they should be removed. There is a pregnancy loss rate from an operation, and it is therefore thought that the early to mid-second trimester (after the fourth month of pregnancy) offers the most opportune time for their removal. Although there is still a chance that the operation may lead to a spontaneous abortion, the danger is minimal compared with that of possible torsion or rupture of the cyst or interruption of later labor and delivery. If the diagnosis of an extrauterine mass is not made until later in the pregnancy, however, it is usually advisable to postpone surgery until term unless there is a high suspicion of cancer.

Notes

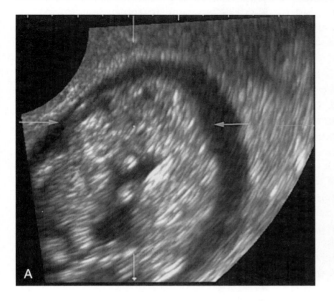

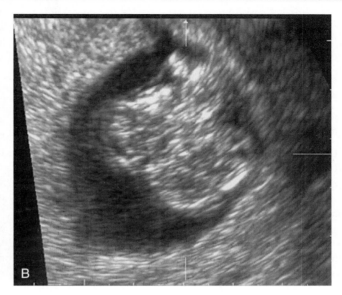

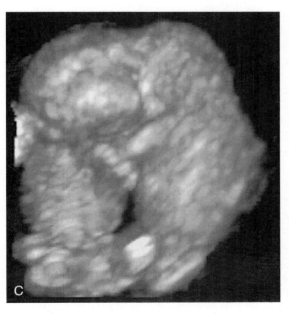

1. A woman presents because of uncertain menstrual dates in the late first trimester for evaluation of embryonic age. What are the findings on this transvaginal examination (Figs. A and B, both three-dimensional [3-D] multiplanar reconstructed images)? Figure A is taken obliquely through the gestational sac, and Figure B is taken through a plane of section at the arrows in Figure A.

2. In the first trimester, what are the ultrasound findings that allow the examiner to determine that a twin gestation is dichorionic-diamniotic (Di-Di)?

3. In the first trimester, the failure to identify an interposed membrane makes the most likely diagnosis of what type of twinning?

4. The detection of conjoined (Siamese) twins raises what possible problems in utero for the twins? For the pregnant woman?

C A S E 2 2

Conjoined (Siamese) Twins in the First Trimester

1. Conjoined (Siamese) twins, joined at the heads.

2. Either two separate sacs, or if the sacs abut one another, a thick (>2 mm) interposed membrane.

3. A monochorionic-monoamniotic (Mono-Mono) twinning.

4. In utero, there are no problems for either the conjoined twins or the pregnant woman. At birth, cesarean section delivery is required.

Acknowledgment

Figures courtesy of Dr. George Bega.

References

Hertzberg BS, Kurtz AB, Choi HY, et al: Significance of membrane thickness in the sonographic evaluation of twin pregnancies. *AJR Am J Roentgenol* 148:151–153, 1987.

Kurtz AB, Wapner RJ, Mata J, et al: Twin pregnancies: Accuracy of first trimester abdominal ultrasound in predicting chorionicity and amnionicity. *Radiology* 185:759–762, 1992.

Cross-Reference

Ultrasound: THE REQUISITES, pp 350–352.

Comment

Most twins (80%) are "fraternal," originating from two separate fertilized ova that develop within separate sacs (their own amniotic and chorionic sacs) and are therefore Di-Di twins. Their ultrasound detection, particularly in the first trimester, is often straightforward: either two separate sacs or a distinct separating (>2 mm) intervening membrane if the sacs impinge on each other. In the first trimester, it is estimated that the accuracy of detection of a Di-Di twinning by transabdominal imaging is approximately 100%; if uncertainty remains, twinning can be detected by a transvaginal study.

In the remaining 20% of twin pregnancies, a single fertilized ovum starts to develop and then splits into "identical" twins of the same gender. If this split occurs before the first day (20% to 30% of cases), the twins develop in completely separate Di-Di sacs similar to true "fraternal" twins.

In the remaining cases of "identical" twins, the fertilized ovum splits later and is enveloped by a single chorion (monochorionic). The twins then share the same environment, either partially (monochorionic-diamniotic [Mono-Di]) or completely (Mono-Mono).

Mono-Di twinning (70% to 75% of identical twins) occurs 1 to 7 days after fertilization. The ultrasound finding of a thin intervening diamniotic membrane is difficult to detect at any time in the pregnancy but is seen most consistently in the first trimester. This may require transvaginal imaging.

In the remaining 1% to 3% of cases of "identical" twins, with the split occurring between days 7 and 13, the twins completely share the same environment. This is a Mono-Mono pregnancy without an intervening membrane. A transvaginal study is needed in the first trimester. Despite the concern that a thin diamniotic membrane may not have been appreciated, the diagnosis of no interposed membrane is fairly accurate. Later in the pregnancy, the diagnosis of a Mono-Mono twinning is less certain.

In rare instances, much less than 1%, the fertilized ovum separates after 13 days. The twins not only share the same sac (Mono-Mono twinning) but also cannot be completely separated, called a conjoined (Siamese) twinning. This most commonly occurs in the thoracic region (thoracopagus). When the thorax and abdominal regions fail to separate, this is called thoracoabdominopagus. Conjoined twins can be joined anywhere from the head (craniopagus) to the pelvis (ischiopagus).

Conjoined twins can share very little or a great deal of their internal structures. Regardless, their in utero development and the woman's welfare, aside from being Mono-Mono twinning with the additional complication of entangled umbilical cords, is unaffected. However, the mode of delivery must be by cesarean section because the overall size of the twins would be too large for vaginal delivery.

The late first-trimester diagnosis of conjoined twins is possible, particularly with transvaginal imaging. To accurately make this diagnosis, not only is it necessary to show that the twins are inseparable (e.g., in Figure A, which suggests that the fetal heads are joined) but also to show that they share internal structures. This is further, but not definitively, shown in Figure B, which shows a scan through the fetal heads. To help further define this case of craniopagus, a 3-D surface imaging reconstruction was performed (Fig. C). All three images make this diagnosis highly likely; however, when doubt remains, it is suggested that the examiner re-examine the pregnancy in the second trimester to confirm the diagnosis and determine the extent of shared internal anatomy.

In this case (see Figs. A to C), 3-D reformatting was important and should be considered whenever the fetal anatomy is difficult to image. The conjoined twins were in an unusual oblique presentation, and standard 2-D images failed to obtain good planes of section. At present, however, the 3-D reconstructed images are not of the same high resolution as 2-D images, although this situation has been gradually improving.

Notes

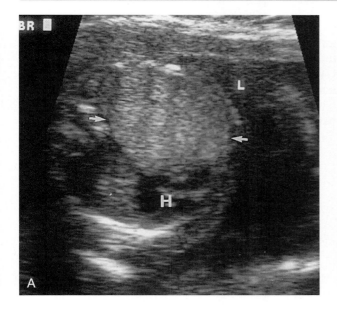

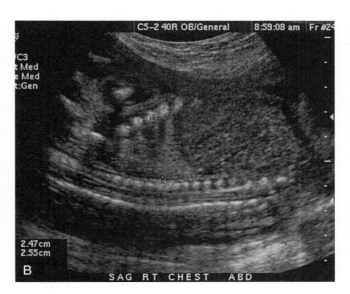

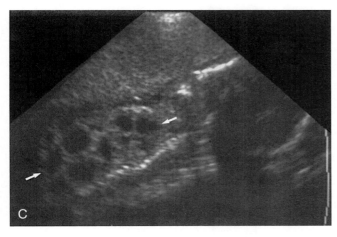

1. Three presentations of the same abnormality are shown in these images of the fetal chest (Fig. A, axial: arrows = an anomaly. H = heart; L = left side of fetus. Fig. B, sagittal: fetal head toward the reader's left. x = an anomaly.) (Fig. C, sagittal: fetal head toward the reader's right. Arrows = an anomaly). What is the diagnosis in these second-trimester fetuses?

2. Which fetal lung masses may appear cystic on a prenatal ultrasound?

3. Which fetal lung masses may have associated anomalies?

4. What predicts the outcome of the neonate with a cystic adenomatoid malformation (CAM)?

Cystic Adenomatoid Malformation

1. CAM type III (see Figs. A and B) and type I (see Fig. C).

2. CAM type I or II, bronchogenic cyst, lobar emphysema, or diaphragmatic hernia containing bowel.

3. CAM type II, extralobar sequestration, and diaphragmatic hernia.

4. Associated anomalies and the amount of residual functioning lung.

Acknowledgment

Figure B, courtesy of Beverly Coleman, MD.

References

Johnson JA, Rumack CM, Johnson ML, et al: Cystic adenomatoid malformation: Antenatal demonstration. *AJR Am J Roentgenol* 142:483–484, 1984.

King SJ, Pilling DW, Walkinshaw S: Fetal echogenic lung lesions: Prenatal ultrasound diagnosis and outcome. *Pediatr Radiol* 25:208–210, 1995.

Cross-Reference

Ultrasound: THE REQUISITES, pp 246–248; 251.

Comment

Congenital CAM is a hamartomatous mass of pulmonary tissue in the lung. It can arise in any lobe of the lung. The classification depends on the size of the cysts. Type I has large cysts (>2 cm), and type II has small cysts. Type III consists of multiple tiny bronchiolar structures and appears as a solid mass. Concomitant renal and gastrointestinal anomalies are present with type II.

On ultrasound, a mass that is cystic (see Fig. C), solid and hyperechoic (see Figs. A and B), or both, can be seen. Type II CAM can also appear solid on prenatal ultrasound if it consists of tiny cysts. In any of these types, the heart and mediastinum may shift (see Fig. A); the cardiac shift and caval compression can result in hydrops. Polyhydramnios is common, probably due to esophageal compression. Detection of a large mass is imperative, because the neonate with a large CAM often has severe respiratory distress necessitating immediate surgery. With large lesions, the outcome depends on the amount of residual functional lung and the presence of associated malformations.

The differential diagnosis of a chest mass depends on the ultrasound characteristics. A solid hyperechoic mass may represent a sequestration, type III CAM, a diaphragmatic hernia containing the liver, or a focal hyperechoic lung due to bronchial obstruction (atresia or mucous plug). A cystic mass could be a type I or II CAM, lobar emphysema, a bronchogenic cyst, or a bowel containing a diaphragmatic hernia.

Detection of any fetal mass warrants a careful search for associated anomalies, present infrequently with extralobar sequestration, and described in association with CAM type II. Close follow-up is required to detect the complication of hydrops if a large mass is present.

Notes

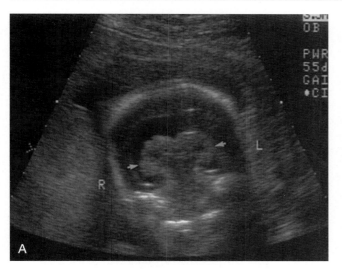
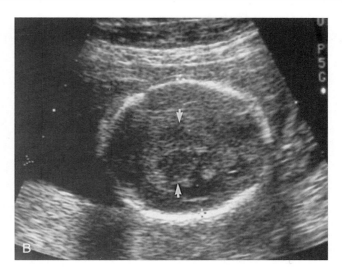

1. What is the spectrum of abnormalities characteristic of the disorder demonstrated by these coronal (Fig. A) and axial (Fig. B) ultrasound images of the fetal brain? Of these, which subtype is shown in this case?

2. Are chromosomal anomalies associated with this disorder?

3. What extracranial malformations have been described in association?

4. What is the prognosis?

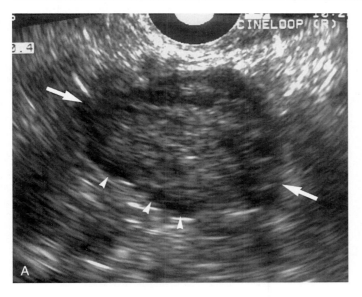
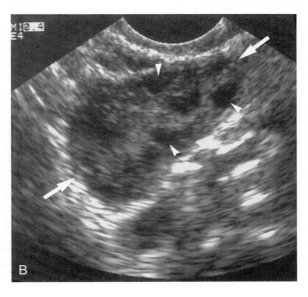

1. This 25-year-old woman presents with infertility. The ultrasound appearance and size of her ovaries (the volume of the right ovary is 18 ml, and that of the left ovary is 14 ml) suggest what diagnosis (Figs. A and B)? What do the arrowheads point to in both images?

2. Is surgery necessary in this type of condition? If not, what is the alternative?

3. Is there an associated syndrome with these ultrasound findings of the ovaries?

4. What are the typical findings in this syndrome, and is the syndrome often present?

Holoprosencephaly

1. Holoprosencephaly: alobar (most severe), semilobar, and lobar (least severe). Alobar.

2. Yes, most commonly trisomy 13.

3. Omphalocele, polydactyly, renal dysplasia, and complex cardiac defects.

4. Dismal, for both alobar and semilobar holoprosencephaly. Variable for the lobar form.

Reference
Nyberg DA, Mack LA, Bronstein A, et al: Holoprosencephaly: Prenatal sonographic diagnosis. *AJR Am J Roentgenol* 149:1050-1058, 1987.

Cross-Reference
Ultrasound: THE REQUISITES, pp 215-216; 235.

Comment
Holoprosencephaly comprises a spectrum of midline brain and facial malformations, due to incomplete cleavage of the forebrain during fetal development. The classification consists of alobar holoprosencephaly (most severe), semilobar (often difficult to distinguish from alobar on prenatal ultrasound), and lobar (least severe). Alobar holoprosencephaly includes a small head, fused thalamus (see Figs. A and B, arrows), a monoventricle, and absence of the corpus callosum, falx cerebri, optic tracts, and olfactory bulbs. Incomplete fusion of the thalami and partial segmentation of the ventricle distinguish semilobar from alobar holoprosencephaly. The most mild form, lobar holoprosencephaly, consists of an absence of optic tracts and olfactory bulbs, similar to septo-optic dysplasia.

The appearance of the ventricular system varies with the severity of the disorder. In alobar holoprosencephaly, there is a monoventricle, with occipital, temporal, and frontal horns absent. Occipital horns may be present in semilobar holoprosencephaly. In the least severe lobar variant, the lateral ventricles are present, but frontal horns do not form.

Chromosomal anomalies and extracranial and facial malformations have all been associated. Approximately 55% of cases have chromosomal anomalies—most commonly trisomy 13. Facial anomalies are more common in the alobar form and include various orbital and nasal malformations ranging from fused orbits with supraorbital proboscis (cyclopia), hypotelorism with midline proboscis (ethmocephaly), hypotelorism, single nostril (cebocephaly), to a medial facial cleft. Extracranial abnormalities described include omphalocele, renal dysplasia, polydactyly, and complex cardiac anomalies.

Notes

Polycystic Ovarian Disease

1. Polycystic ovaries. Multiple small peripherally placed follicles.

2. No, fertility medication, particularly clomiphene citrate (Clomid), may cause successful ovulation and pregnancy.

3. Yes, Stein-Leventhal syndrome.

4. Hirsutism, infertility, and polycystic ovaries. No—the entire syndrome is not typically present.

References
Hann LE, Hall DA, McArdle CR, Seibel M: Polycystic ovarian disease: Sonographic spectrum. *Radiology* 150:531-534, 1984.

Yeh HS, Futterweit W, Thornton JC: Polycystic ovarian disease: US features in 104 patients. *Radiology* 163:111-116, 1987.

Cross-Reference
Ultrasound: THE REQUISITES, pp 396-397

Comment
Polycystic ovarian disease (PCOD) has a spectrum of findings, both sonographic and clinically. Polycystic ovaries (PCOs) can be detected incidentally in normally fertile women without additional problems. The most common ovarian feature is multiple small follicles between 5 and 8 mm in size, typically peripherally located (see Figs. A and B, arrowheads). The classic appearance of PCOs is that of rounded enlarged ovaries, commonly greater then 15 ml in volume (length × width × height ÷ 2). However, PCOs may be normal in size, ovoid instead of round, and not enlarged.

The clinical significance of PCOs is based on clinical symptomatology and laboratory findings.

Although PCOs may be incidentally noted, without clinical or physical examination findings, they can also be associated with various clinical and laboratory findings. The full-blown clinical syndrome is hirsutism, infertility, and oligomenorrhea, and it is then called Stein-Leventhal syndrome. In these cases, there are frequently abnormal serum antigens or an increased luteinizing hormone/follicle-stimulating hormone ratio.

PCOs are known pathologically to have fibrous capsules. As a result, past treatment had been a surgical wedge resection of the ovary to disrupt this capsule. With the advent of fertility medicines, however, in particular clomiphene citrate, the treatment has become hormonal.

Notes

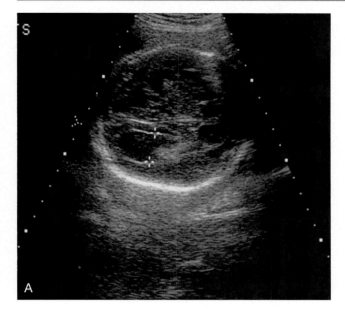

1. In this second-trimester fetal head, the atrium of the lateral ventricles measures 12 mm (Fig. A, +'s). What is the normal range of size for the atrium of the lateral ventricle?

2. List three causes of hydrocephalus.

3. Is there an association of hydrocephalus with other central nervous system (CNS) or systemic malformations?

4. Does postnatal ventricular shunting benefit noncommunicating or communicating hydrocephalus?

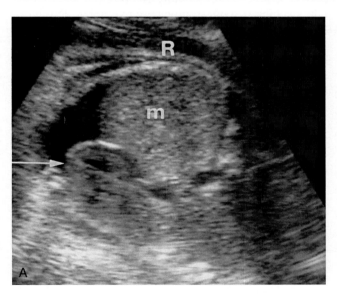
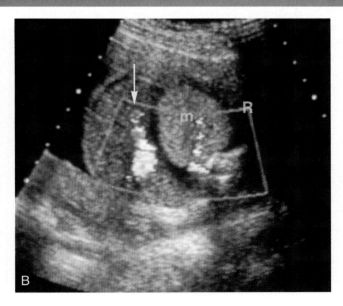

1. What is the most likely diagnosis of the thoracic mass (m) shown in these axial images of the fetal chest (Figs. A and B)? Figure B is a color Doppler image of A. (Arrow = heart; R = right side of the fetus.)

2. How does color Doppler imaging help in making the diagnosis of sequestration?

3. Are there any anomalies associated with sequestrations?

4. Where are sequestrations typically located?

CASE 26

Hydrocephalus

1. 4 to 8 mm (up to 10 mm).

2. Aqueductal stenosis, Arnold-Chiari malformation, mass (rare).

3. Yes, CNS malformations, systemic malformations, and chromosomal anomalies.

4. Obstructive or noncommunicating hydrocephalus.

References

Hertzberg BS, Kliewer MA, Bowie JD: Fetal cerebral ventriculomegaly: Misidentification of the true medial boundary of the ventricle at ultrasound. *Radiology* 205:813–816, 1997.

Hilpert PL, Hall BE, Kurtz AB: The atria of the fetal lateral ventricles: A sonographic study of normal atrial size and choroid plexus volume. *AJR Am J Roentgenol* 164:731–734, 1995.

Cross-Reference

Ultrasound: THE REQUISITES, pp 210–214, 234.

Comment

Fetal hydrocephalus can be diagnosed with prenatal ultrasound by detecting an enlarged atrium of the lateral ventricle. The upper limits of normal is 8 mm before 25 weeks' gestation and 10 mm later in the gestation. The normal choroid plexus should fill 50% to 60% of the lateral ventricle. In the setting of hydrocephalus, choroid is surrounded by fluid within the dilated ventricle and appears to dangle, an important secondary sign.

Care must be taken to obtain an accurate measurement of the lateral ventricle. The atrium must be measured perpendicularly at the edge of the choroid plexus. False enlargement can be diagnosed if the interface with the subarachnoid space is misinterpreted as the lateral border of the ventricle; additionally, the medial boundary of the cerebral hemisphere must not be mistaken for the medial border of the lateral ventricle. Typically, the lateral ventricle further from the transducer is better seen, whereas the closer ventricle is obscured by reverberation artifact from the overlying calvarium (Fig. A).

The etiology of hydrocephalus may be difficult to determine in utero. Aqueductal stenosis presents with enlarged third and lateral ventricles, but a small fourth ventricle. Arnold-Chiari malformation consists of a myelomeningocele, a small posterior fossa, and associated ventriculomegaly as well as a lemon-shaped skull early in the gestation. An obstructing mass is an uncommon cause of fetal hydrocephalus.

Notes

CASE 27

Sequestration

1. Diagnosis = sequestration.

2. Identification of a systemic feeding artery.

3. Infrequently with the extralobar type.

4. Lower lobe; left greater than right.

References

Bromley B, Parad R, Estroff JA, Benacerraf BR: Fetal lung masses: Prenatal course and outcome. *J Ultrasound Med* 14:927–936, 1995.

Felker RE, Tonkin IL: Imaging of pulmonary sequestration. *AJR Am J Roentgenol* 154:241–249, 1990.

Hernanz-Schulman M, Stein SM, Neblett WW, et al: Pulmonary sequestration: Diagnosis with color Doppler sonography and new theory of associated hydrothorax. *Radiology* 180:817–821, 1991.

Cross-Reference

Ultrasound: THE REQUISITES, p 247.

Comment

Pulmonary sequestration is defined as a portion of the lung that receives systemic rather than pulmonary arterial supply and is separated from the tracheobronchial tree. Intralobar sequestration is most common, contained within the normal pleura. Extralobar sequestration has its own pleura. Because intralobar sequestrations present in infants older than 2 months, many believe it is an acquired entity. Accordingly, most prenatally diagnosed sequestrations are extralobar. Extralobar sequestrations can be located between the lower lobe and the hemidiaphragm, within the diaphragm or lung, in the pleural or pericardial space, and even in the retroperitoneum. Most occur on the left side. Both intralobar and extralobar sequestrations have systemic arterial supply, usually from the aorta.

Extralobar sequestration has previously been reported to be associated with diaphragmatic hernia and other anomalies, including complex congenital heart disease. However, these associations are now considered to be very infrequent.

Prenatal ultrasound shows a supradiaphragmatic or infradiaphragmatic hyperechoic mass, usually on the left side. Mediastinal and cardiac shift will result if the sequestration is large (see Fig. A). In some cases, as the fetus grows, the sequestration becomes relatively smaller. Blood flow may be evident with color Doppler imaging, and in some cases systemic arterial supply may be visible from the aorta (see Fig. B). Polyhydramnios may be present. Rarely, tension hydrothorax and hydrops may occur and are believed to result from torsion of the sequestration (see Fig. A, anterior to the heart).

Notes

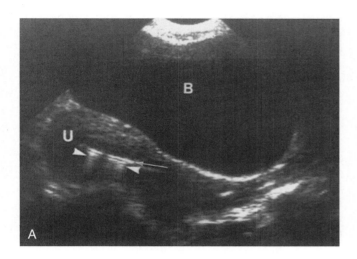

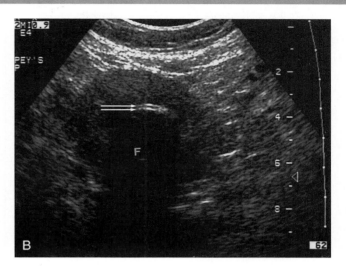

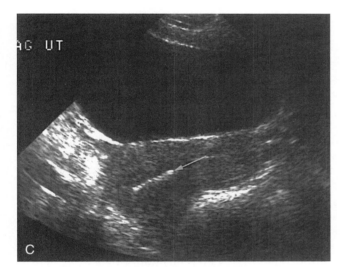

1. A 35-year-old woman with a previously inserted intrauterine contraceptive device (IUCD) presents for ultrasound of the uterus because her physical examination failed to identify the IUCD string within the vagina. Figure A is an ultrasound sagittal transabdominal scan. What are the intrauterine findings, and to what are the arrow and arrowheads pointing? (U = uterus; B = urinary bladder.)

2. What is the role of ultrasound in the evaluation of an IUCD?

3. On physical examination of the pelvis, if the string is not identified, what are the three diagnostic possibilities?

4. Are IUCDs commonly used at present in the United States?

Intrauterine Contraceptive Device

1. An IUCD well positioned within the endometrial canal. The arrow points to the IUCD; the arrowheads point to reverberation artifacts from the metal in the IUCD.

2. To evaluate for the intrauterine presence and position of the IUCD.

3. The IUCD is in correct position, but the string has pulled back into the cervical or uterine canal. The IUCD has been expelled along with the string. The IUCD has partially or completely perforated the uterine wall and the string has, therefore, been pulled up into the uterine canal or into or through the myometrium.

4. No.

Reference
Copeland LJ: *Textbook of Gynecology*. Philadelphia, WB Saunders, 1993, pp 164-169.

Cross-Reference
Ultrasound: THE REQUISITES, pp 373-375.

Comment
IUCDs have been used since the early 1900s to prevent pregnancy. Initially, silkworm gut was inserted in the uterine cavity. Since then, IUCDs have been steadily refined, and today many types of IUCD are available. IUCDs are better suited for older women who have been previously pregnant. Younger IUCD users experience higher pregnancy rates and more expulsions, and they have them removed more frequently for medical reasons. Contraindications to use of an IUCD include pregnancy, a history of pelvic inflammatory disease, undiagnosed vaginal bleeding, uterine anomalies, and large fibroid tumors. Primarily for these reasons, IUCD usage has significantly decreased in the United States.

IUCDs have a number of different ultrasound appearances, depending on their shape and composition. They use thin plastic tubing, metal wrapping, or a combination of both. A Copper 7, for example, has a long arm of wrapped copper along the long axis of the uterus and a small arm of plastic in transaxial view in the upper body or fundus. The metal wrapping exhibits a "reverberation artifact," a series of parallel lines that get weaker and weaker from the IUCD posteriorly (see Fig. A) when the IUCD is parallel to the ultrasound beam. The plastic tubing presents as two parallel lines, an entrance and an exit echo, which are shown in a second case (Fig. B, an axial image of the uterine fundus. Arrows = two parallel lines). A hypoechoic solid mass (F = fibroid) is posterior in the uterine fundus and is displacing the IUCD anteriorly.

Ultrasound is very accurate in detecting an IUCD when it is correctly positioned. When the uterus is normal and there is no distortion of the endometrial canal, the IUCD has a midline position. However, with an IUCD in place, the thickness of the endometrial complex is difficult to evaluate. When fibroids or a retroverted or retroflexed uterus (typically a globular-appearing uterus) are present, the determination of the exact position of the IUCD in relation to the endometrial complex may become difficult (Fig. C, arrow; see also Fig. B). In Figure C, which shows an ultrasound sagittal image of a retroverted uterus, the long arm of the Copper 7 is well positioned within the uterus. Reverberation artifacts are not present, because the IUCD is not parallel to the ultrasound beam. Fibroids may change the position of the uterine cavity so that the IUCD may appear to be partially perforating the uterine wall. In general, plain radiographs are not useful, because a distorted position on ultrasound would also appear distorted on plain films. For a more definitive imaging study, a hysterosalpingogram and, more recently, a sonohysterogram would be useful. At present neither magnetic resonance imaging nor computed tomography has been used for IUCD positioning but would be considered in technically difficult cases.

One of the most common clinical uses of ultrasound in the evaluation of IUCDs is to determine whether the IUCD is still present within the uterus when the string is no longer present on pelvic examination. Because of the potential for expulsion and the potential for perforation either into or through the uterine wall, failure to detect a string within the vagina often leads to an ultrasound examination. If the IUCD is well positioned within the uterus, then the retracted string is of no consequence. Conversely, the failure to detect an IUCD is often an accurate determination of expulsion. When clinical symptomatology still makes a consideration of perforation likely, the negative uterine study does not entirely rule out perforation, and a plain anteroposterior radiograph of the pelvis will detect the perforated radiopaque IUCD.

IUCDs have complications. In addition to unexpected pregnancies, infections are more common. Although typically bacterial, there may also be fungal infections including actinomycosis. Expulsion may also occur. If a pregnancy occurs after implantation of an IUCD, the role of ultrasound is to detect whether it is still present. The IUCD does not create a risk to the pregnancy, because it is in the endometrial cavity and is not within the chorionic sac. However, if on physical examination, the string is still projecting into the vagina, the cervical plug will not form and there is a potential for an ascending infection. The IUCD should then be removed, often under ultrasound guidance.

Notes

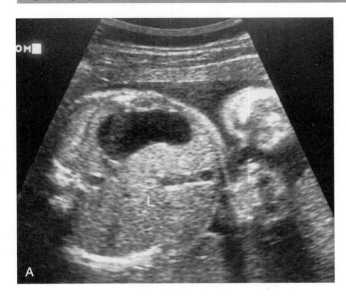

1. What is this cystic structure in the left upper quadrant in this second-trimester fetus (Fig. A, axial image of the upper abdomen. L = liver)? Is it enlarged?

2. Name a potential cause of a distended stomach.

3. When is the stomach reliably visualized?

4. When does the fetus begin swallowing?

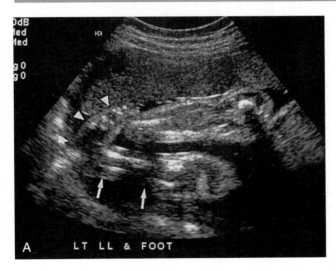

1. In this 27-week-old fetus, what is the finding on this image of its left leg (Fig. A)? Arrows denote the lower leg; arrowheads denote the foot.

2. What percentage of cases are bilateral?

3. Are chromosomal anomalies associated?

4. Name two extrinsic causes of this entity.

Enlarged Fetal Stomach

1. Stomach. Yes.

2. Duodenal atresia.

3. By 19 weeks.

4. 11 gestational weeks.

References

Blaas HG, Eik-Nes SH, Kiserud T, Hellevik LR: Early development of the abdominal wall, stomach and heart from 7 to 12 weeks of gestation: A longitudinal ultrasound study. *Ultrasound Obstet Gynecol* 6:240–249, 1995.

Ozmen MN, Onderoglu L, Ciftci AO, et al: Prenatal diagnosis of gastric duplication cyst. *J Ultrasound Med* 16:219–222, 1997.

Zimmer EZ, Chao CR, Abramovich G, Timor-Tritsch IE: Fetal stomach measurements: Not reproducible by the same observer. *J Ultrasound Med* 11:663–665, 1992.

Cross-Reference

Ultrasound: THE REQUISITES, pp 253–258.

Comment

Visualization of a normal fetal stomach is important to exclude esophageal disease, cardiovascular disease as well as gastric and small bowel anomalies. The fetal stomach should be seen in normal patients by 19 weeks; one series using transvaginal ultrasound demonstrated gastric visualization in all normal cases by 11 weeks. The location and size of the stomach are specific criteria that are assessed in utero. An abnormal location, with regard to the heart, is an indicator of cardiovascular disease.

Charts are available for reference describing the normal mean gastric size at any gestational age. Because the stomach is dynamic, measurements are difficult to reproduce reliably in normal patients. The fetus initiates swallowing movements at 11 weeks. As early as 14 weeks' gestational age, the stomach can be shown to fill and empty. A small or absent stomach can be seen with several abnormalities, including esophageal atresia, oligohydramnios, and central nervous system or neck malformations that prevent swallowing.

Enlargement of the fetal stomach (see Fig. A) is a less well known potential sign of abnormality. It has been described in cases of duodenal atresia. The differential diagnosis of a cystic mass in the region of the stomach includes the rare gastric duplication cyst. These cysts occur most commonly along the greater curvature and do not usually communicate with the stomach; thus they remain fixed in size.

Notes

Clubfoot

1. Clubfoot.

2. Slightly more than half.

3. Yes.

4. Oligohydramnios and amniotic band syndrome.

References

Benacerraf BR, Frigoletto TD: Prenatal ultrasound diagnosis of clubfoot. *Radiology* 155:211–213, 1985.

Hashimoto BE, Filly RA, Callen PW: Sonographic diagnosis of clubfoot in utero. *J Ultrasound Med* 5:81–83, 1986.

Shipp TD, Benacerraf BR: The significance of prenatally identified isolated clubfoot: Is amniocentesis indicated? *Am J Obstet Gynecol* 178:600–602, 1998.

Cross-Reference

Ultrasound: The REQUISITES, p 305.

Comment

Clubfoot is a common congenital anomaly that occurs bilaterally in slightly more than half of the cases. Many cases are familial, and the risk is as high as 25% if the parent has a clubfoot. Although the most common cause is idiopathic, associated abnormalities warrant a careful search with prenatal ultrasound once clubfoot is detected.

Clubfoot is associated with chromosomal anomalies, such as trisomy 13 and trisomy 18. Even if the prenatal sonogram fails to detect other malformations, the incidence of karyotype abnormality is 6%.

In addition to chromosomal anomalies, clubfoot deformity is associated with other malformations in 10% of cases. Cleft lip and palate, micrognathia, facial deformities, congenital heart disease, and hip dislocations are among the associated anomalies. Neurologic abnormalities associated with clubfoot include meningomyelocele and hydrocephalus. Numerous congenital syndromes and musculoskeletal disorders include clubfoot in the spectrum of anomalies: Gordon's syndrome (camptodactyly and cleft palate), distal arthrogryposis (fixated hands and feet), nail-patella syndrome, muscular dystrophies, and Pierre Robin syndrome (congenital heart disease). Extrinsic causes can also lead to clubfoot deformity, including oligohydramnios and amniotic band syndrome.

The ultrasound appearance relies on an unusual configuration between the foot and the lower leg (see Fig. A). Once seen, careful evaluation of the other extremities for bilaterality and clubhands should be undertaken. The more the limbs are affected, the greater is the possibility of a congenital syndrome or a musculoskeletal disorder.

Notes

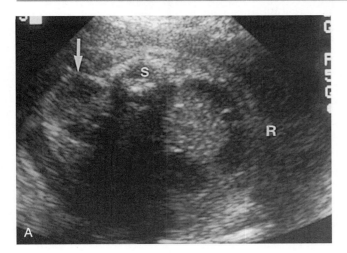

1. What does the arrow point to in this mid-abdominal axial image of a second-trimester fetus, and what is the abnormal finding (Fig. A)? What are possible etiologies? (S = spine; R = toward the fetal right.)

2. What are the three criteria for prenatal ultrasound diagnosis if this anomaly is bilateral?

3. How early can the diagnosis be made?

4. How can color Doppler be useful?

Renal Agenesis

1. The arrow points to the normal left kidney. The right kidney is not in its usually paraspinal location. Possible etiologies are unilateral renal agenesis, ectopically placed kidney such as a pelvic kidney, or crossed fused ectopia.

2. If bilateral, in addition to the absence of the kidneys, the urinary bladder is not visualized and oligohydramnios is present.

3. Early second trimester (12 to 13 weeks).

4. It can identify the abdominal aorta by its flow, even when severe oligohydramnios is present, and can confirm absence of renal arterial flow to the suspected side.

References

Mackenzie FM, Kingston GO, Oppenheimer L: The early prenatal diagnosis of bilateral renal agenesis using transvaginal sonography and color Doppler ultrasonography. *J Ultrasound Med* 13:49–51, 1994.

Sherer DM, Thompson HO, Armstrong B, Woods JR: Prenatal sonographic diagnosis of fetal renal agenesis. *J Clin Ultrasound* 18:648–652, 1990.

Cross-Reference

Ultrasound: THE REQUISITES, pp 75, 279–280.

Comment

The fetal kidneys can be seen as early as 12 to 14 weeks. By 12 weeks, the urinary bladder can be seen in approximately half of cases. Renal agenesis can be unilateral (see Fig. A) or bilateral; the latter case is fatal (Potter's syndrome). Autopsy studies report the incidence of unilateral agenesis to be 1 in 400, and bilateral agenesis to be 1 in 2653. Bilateral renal agenesis is an autosomal recessive condition.

Routine prenatal sonography requires the identification of both fetal kidneys. On an axial image of the fetal mid-abdomen, both kidneys should be detected on the same image. If one is not visualized, as in this case (see Fig. A), the abnormal renal region should be evaluated. Occasionally, bowel with peristalsis can be seen. The adrenal glands, however, are much more prominent in utero and are up to one third of the size of the kidneys. To the casual observer, when unilateral (or bilateral) renal agenesis occurs, the adrenal glands, which are discoid and of the same echogenicity as the kidneys, can fill the renal beds and mimic the kidneys.

If it can be established that one kidney is not in its normal position, an ectopic location should be sought. In particular, the fetal pelvis should be examined for a pelvic kidney. The normal side should be further examined for a possible cross-fused ectopia. If unilateral agen- esis is confirmed, the contralateral kidney should also be carefully inspected to exclude other genitourinary anomalies such as an associated multicystic dysplastic kidney. Additional associated anomalies include congenital uterine anomalies in females and seminal vesicle cysts and cryptorchidism in males.

In unilateral renal agenesis, the amniotic fluid remains normal. Bilateral renal agenesis leads to marked oligohydramnios, which results in pulmonary hypoplasia in utero. This condition is incompatible with life. The urinary bladder is not visualized (or appears to be very small), and the stomach may be secondarily small or absent due to oligohydramnios. The ultrasound examination becomes technically difficult in the setting of severe oligohydramnios. Doppler ultrasound has proved helpful in confirming the absence of renal artery flow bilaterally.

Notes

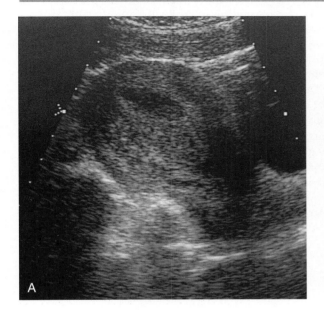

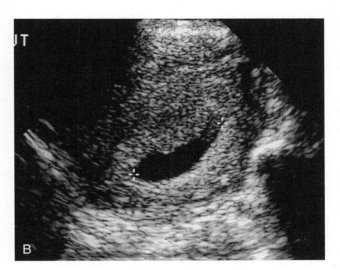

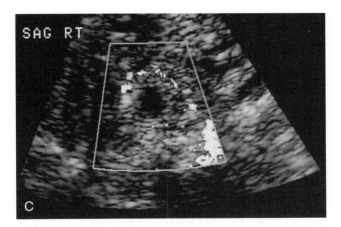

1. What accounts for the ultrasound finding in this first-trimester examination (Fig. A, transabdominal of the uterus; Fig. B, transvaginal of the uterus; and Fig. C, color Doppler image of the right adnexa)?

2. What is the intradecidual sign?

3. What is the double decidual reaction?

4. What is the significance of decidual cysts?

Ectopic Pregnancy

1. Right ectopic pregnancy with an intrauterine pseudogestational sac.

2. The early intrauterine sac is situated adjacent to or abutting the uterine cavity and is embedded in the decidua.

3. Two concentric hyperechoic rings that surround the early intrauterine gestational sac.

4. Indicate decidual breakdown.

References

Ackerman TE, Levi CS, Lyons EA, et al: Decidual cyst: Endovaginal sonographic sign of ectopic pregnancy. *Radiology* 189:727–731, 1993.

Laing FC, Brown DL, Price JF, et al: Intradecidual sign: Is it effective in diagnosis of early intrauterine pregnancy? *Radiology* 204:655–660, 1997.

Parvey HR, Dubinsky TJ, Johnston DA, Maklad NF: The chorionic rim and low impedance intrauterine arterial flow in the detection of early intrauterine pregnancy. *AJR Am J Roentgenol* 167:1479–1485, 1996.

Cross-Reference

Ultrasound: THE REQUISITES, pp 415–431.

Comment

Detection of a true intrauterine gestational sac is paramount to the exclusion of an ectopic pregnancy. Intraendometrial fluid collections, also known as "decidual casts," should not be misinterpreted as a gestational sac. It is often called a pseudogestational sac (see Figs. A and B). These collections can be seen in the setting of an ectopic pregnancy and are caused by the hormonal influence of the ectopic pregnancy. Several characteristics of a true early intrauterine gestational sac have been shown to be helpful in distinguishing this from intraendometrial fluid when the intrauterine pregnancy (IUP) is visualized before the development of a yolk sac or fetal pole.

Before the double decidual sac becomes apparent, the location of the sac is an important criterion. The "intradecidual sign" refers to a sac located adjacent to or abutting the endometrial lining, embedded within the decidual reaction. The decidual cast or intraendometrial fluid, which is seen in cases of ectopic pregnancies, is located within the uterine cavity. Unfortunately, this sign has been shown to have low sensitivity and specificity.

The double decidual reaction refers to two concentric hyperechoic rings that surround the early intrauterine gestatational sac. Unfortunately, this sign may not be present with a normal intrauterine gestational sac. The chorionic rim, a hyperechoic rim bordering an intrauterine collection of fluid, has been shown to be a more sensitive indicator of an IUP, particularly if there is an associated high diastolic flow. Although color Doppler imaging can be used, care must be taken to avoid using pulsed Doppler on or near a normal early embryo.

Decidual cysts are 1- to 5-mm diameter simple cysts that are located in the decidual reaction and are remote from the endometrial canal. They may be found at the junction of the endometrium and myometrium. They do not have a hyperechoic trophoblastic ring and are believed to represent an early breakdown of the decidua.

Notes

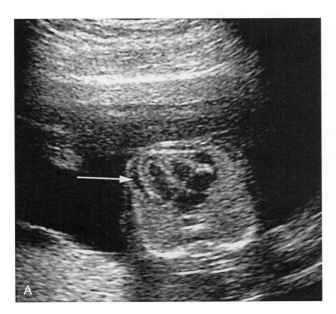
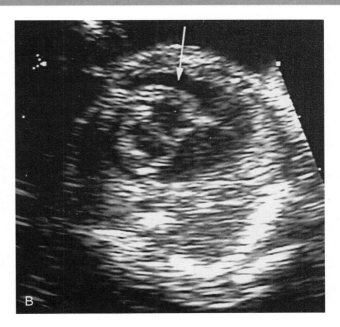

1. What is the finding (denoted by an arrow) on these images of the fetal chest (Figs. A and B)?
2. What percentage of normal fetuses have minimal pericardial fluid in the second trimester?
3. What amount of pericardial fluid is considered to be normal in these fetuses?
4. What viruses may cause fetal pericardial fluid?

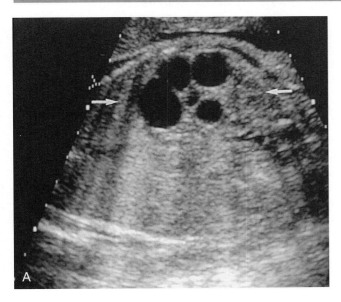

1. What is the most likely diagnosis and the differential diagnoses of the abnormality (Fig. A, arrows) adjacent to the spine on this sagittal view of the fetal abdomen?
2. Why is it important to evaluate the other kidney?
3. Is there any risk of malignant degeneration of a multicystic dysplastic kidney (MCDK) postnatally?
4. What is the typical outcome of an MCDK?

Pericardial Effusion

1. Pericardial effusions, Figure A is small; Figure B is moderate in size.

2. Greater than 70%.

3. Up to 2 mm.

4. Maternal parvovirus, cytomegalovirus (CMV), and human immunodeficiency virus (HIV).

Acknowledgment

Figures for Case 33 courtesy of Mr. Dennis Wood.

References

Di Salvo DN, Brown DL, Doubilet PM, et al: Clinical significance of isolated fetal pericardial effusion. *J Ultrasound Med* 13:291-293, 1994.

Dizon-Townson DS, Dildy GA, Clark SL: A prospective evaluation of fetal pericardial fluid in 506 second-trimester low-risk pregnancies. *Obstet Gynecol* 90:958-961, 1997.

Sharland G, Lockhart S: Isolated pericardial effusion: An indication for fetal karyotyping? *Ultrasound Obstet Gynecol* 6:29-32, 1995.

Cross-Reference

Ultrasound: THE REQUISITES, pp 243-245.

Comment

A small amount of pericardial fluid is normal in the second trimester. A study of more than 500 low-risk pregnancies demonstrated that between 16 and 25 weeks of gestation, a small quantity of pericardial fluid (defined as 2 mm or less) is a normal finding detected in 71% of the cases.

Larger quantities of pericardial fluid can be associated with additional abnormalities. Structural cardiac anomalies and arrhythmias must be excluded with fetal echocardiography. Fetuses with hydrops can have pericardial effusions. Viral causes have been reported, most commonly parvovirus, CMV, and HIV. Intrauterine growth restriction has also been associated.

If the pericardial effusion is determined to be the only abnormality, the outcome is controversial. One study demonstrated that fetuses with isolated significant pericardial effusion had a higher incidence of chromosomal anomalies (31%), particularly Down syndrome. However, a separate study demonstrated that 52 fetuses with pericardial effusions, ranging from 2 to 7 mm in thickness, had no significant difference in outcome compared with all neonates born during the same period.

Notes

Multicystic Dysplastic Kidney

1. MCDK is the most likely diagnosis. Differential diagnoses are hydronephrosis, cystic mesoblastic nephroma, and a rare cystic Wilms' tumor.

2. Contralateral renal anomalies occur in 40%.

3. Yes.

4. The kidney usually regresses.

References

De Oliveira-Filho AG, Carvalho MH, Sbragia-Neto L, et al: Wilms' tumor in a prenatally diagnosed multicystic dysplastic kidney. *J Urol* 158:1926-1927, 1997.

Minevich E, Wacksman J, Phipps L, et al: The importance of accurate diagnosis and early close follow-up in patients with suspected multicystic dysplastic kidney. *J Urol* 158:1301-1304, 1997.

Cross-Reference

Ultrasound: THE REQUISITES, pp 283-284.

Comment

Pathologically, a multicystic dysplastic kidney is replaced by noncommunicating cysts of varying sizes, comprised of dilated collecting tubules. The etiology is believed to be either an obstruction during embryogenesis or primary dysplasia due to abnormalities of metanephric blastema and ureteral bud.

MCDK is often diagnosed with prenatal ultrasound; it can present as an abdominal mass in the neonate. The differential diagnosis of a multicystic renal mass in the fetus includes hydronephrosis (in which the cystic areas communicate), cystic mesoblastic nephroma (the most common neonatal genitourinary neoplasm), and cystic Wilms' tumor.

On prenatal ultrasound, the kidney is replaced by multiple simple cysts. In utero, growth of the dysplastic tissue can cause an MCDK to enlarge, warranting follow-up ultrasound examinations. Careful evaluation of the contralateral functioning kidney is essential, because additional congenital renal anomalies occur in up to 40% of cases. Contralateral MCDK (a lethal condition) comprises half of these, with ureteropelvic junction obstruction and renal agenesis accounting for the remaining 20%. Contralateral reflux is also common.

MCDK regresses with increasing age postnatally. Complications include hypertension, which is uncommon, and malignant degeneration, which is rare. Both Wilms' tumor and renal cell carcinoma have been described arising from an MCDK. Close follow-up is recommended; some physicians advocate surgical removal of the kidney.

Notes

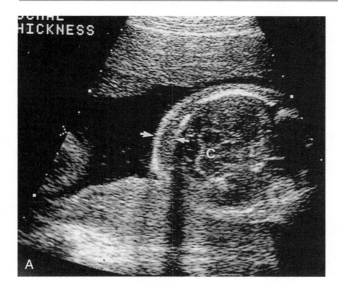

1. What is the soft tissue abnormality (arrows) posterior to the occiput in this 20-week-old fetus (Fig. A; C = cerebellum). What is the most commonly associated karyotype abnormality?

2. What constitutes nuchal thickening?

3. At what age do most women have a fetus with this disorder?

4. What serum screening test is used, and what is the sensitivity?

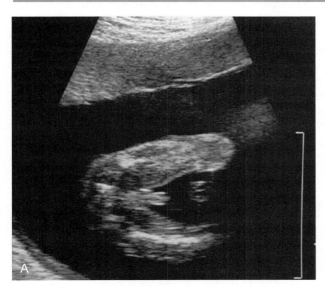

1. In addition to the gender of this fetus, what does this image reveal (Fig. A)?

2. What are two common fetal organ systems that have anomalies associated with this condition?

3. What renal mass is associated?

4. Is there an increased incidence of chromosomal anomalies?

Trisomy 21 (Down syndrome)—Basic

1. Nuchal skin thickening. Trisomy 21 (Down syndrome).

2. Nuchal translucency (thickness) greater than 3 mm in the first trimester or greater than 6 mm between 16 and 22 weeks.

3. Most cases occur in women younger than 35 years of age.

4. The triple screen measures maternal serum α-fetoprotein (AFP), estradiol, and β-human chorionic gonadotropin (HCG). Its sensitivity for Down syndrome is 60%.

References

Benacerraf BR: Use of sonographic markers to determine the risk of Down syndrome in second trimester fetuses. *Radiology* 201:619-620, 1996.

Rotmensch S, Liberati M, Bronshtein M, et al: Prenatal sonographic findings in 187 fetuses with Down syndrome. *Prenat Diagn* 17:1001-1009, 1997.

Cross-Reference

Ultrasound: THE REQUISITES, pp 221, 295.

Comment

Down syndrome, or trisomy 21, is the most common chromosomal anomaly diagnosed in newborns. Although advanced maternal age is a known risk factor, most cases occur in women younger than 35 years of age. The maternal serum triple screen of AFP, estradiol, and β-HCG, which is obtained at 15 weeks, has a sensitivity of only 60% for detection of Down syndrome.

Ultrasound can detect a number of normal anatomic variants as well as malformations associated with Down syndrome. Sensitivity for prenatal detection is as high as 80% using these markers. Nuchal translucency (thickening) greater than 3 mm in the first trimester or greater than 6 mm between 16 and 22 weeks (see Fig. A) carries an increased risk of aneuploidy, most commonly trisomy 21. A short humerus and femur, dilatation of the renal pelves, and hyperechogenic (echogenic) bowel may also be present, and a combination of findings makes the diagnosis more certain.

Additional associated malformations, which can be detected prenatally, include cystic hygroma, duodenal atresia, and hydrocephalus, as well as cardiac abnormalities (atrioventricular canal, ventricular septal defect, tetralogy of Fallot, and transposition of the great vessels).

Ultrasound *may* appear normal in the setting of Down syndrome. Conversely, any abnormal finding does not definitively make the diagnosis of Down syndrome.

Notes

Polyhydramnios

1. Polyhydramnios.

2. Gastrointestinal (GI) and central nervous system.

3. Mesoblastic nephroma.

4. Yes.

Reference

Barnhard Y, Bar-Hava I, Divon MY: Is polyhydramnios in an ultrasonographically normal fetus an indication for genetic evaluation. *Am J Obstet Gynecol* 173:1523-1527, 1995.

Cross-Reference

Ultrasound: THE REQUISITES, pp 208, 210.

Comment

Polyhydramnios, shown in this case, may not present until after 24 weeks. The causes include maternal, fetal, and placental abnormalities. The quantity of fluid can be an indicator of the cause. Mild increases in amniotic fluid are often idiopathic. Larger volumes of fluid more commonly indicate the presence of an anomaly. The ability to make the diagnosis on this one image emphasizes the importance of subjective evaluation of the fluid volume; in addition, the amniotic fluid index (AFI) can be calculated and compared with the range of normal for the specific gestational age.

Fetal anomalies are present in approximately 12% to 20% of cases. These relate to the inability of the fetus to swallow the amniotic fluid or an obstruction to the passage of amniotic fluid through the GI tract. Central nervous system malformations such as anencephaly, encephalocele, and Dandy-Walker malformation can cause decreased swallowing. Esophageal atresia and duodenal atresia result in a GI obstruction. Thoracic masses that obstruct the esophagus, such as a large congenital cystic adenomatoid malformation or diaphragmatic hernia, will result in polyhydramnios. Fetal hydrops that develops from any cause is another etiology.

Fetal masses can present with secondary polyhydramnios. These masses include head, neck, and sacrococcygeal teratoma. Several unusual associations include mesoblastic nephroma and a large fetal ovarian cyst.

Fetal chromosomal anomalies are present in 4% of cases. This should be suspected if specific associated fetal anomalies are documented or if the fetus develops intrauterine growth retardation.

Certain causes may not be apparent on prenatal sonography, including maternal diabetes mellitus or infection (the cause in this case) triggered by cytomegalovirus or toxoplasmosis.

Notes

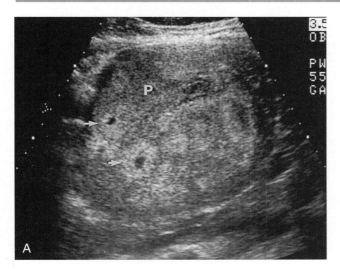

1. What is the differential diagnosis of these lesions (arrows) within the placenta (P) (Fig. A)?
2. Which lesion occurs more commonly on the maternal side of the placenta?
3. Which laboratory abnormality is associated with several of these entities?
4. What is the typical ultrasound appearance of a placental infarct?

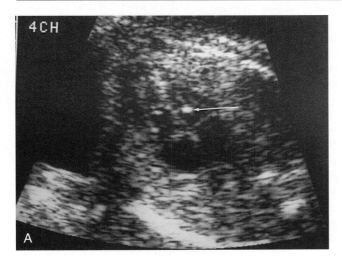

1. In this four-chamber image of the fetal heart, what is the finding denoted by an arrow in the left ventricle (Fig. A)?
2. What is the incidence in fetuses with Down syndrome?
3. What is the hyperechoic focus pathologically?
4. Does the side of the heart (right versus left ventricle) where the calcification is seen have prognostic significance?

Placental Infarct

1. Placental infarct, intervillous thrombus, fibrin deposition, and (less likely) hematoma.

2. Infarct.

3. Elevated α-fetoprotein (AFP).

4. Many are nonvisualized; hypoechoic or echogenic.

References

Harris RD, Simpson WA, Pet LR, et al: Placental hypo-echoic/anechoic areas and infarction: Sonographic-pathologic correlation. *Radiology* 176:75–90, 1990.

Levine AB, Frieden FJ, Stein JL, Pisnanont P: Prenatal sonographic diagnosis of placental infarction in association with elevated maternal serum alpha-fetoprotein. *J Ultrasound Med* 3:169–171, 1993.

Cross-Reference

Ultrasound: THE REQUISITES, pp 335, 337.

Comment

Small placental infarcts, as shown in this case (see Fig. A), are not uncommon and occur in approximately 25% of pregnancies. Larger infarcts are associated with complications including intrauterine growth retardation (IUGR) and increased perinatal mortality. These infarcts are more common in pregnancies complicated with preeclampsia or in women with essential hypertension. Placental infarcts are associated with an elvated maternal AFP.

The ultrasound appearance of a placental infarct has been described in several studies, and the descriptions vary. Harris and associates reported that placental infarcts are not visible with ultrasound unless they are complicated by hemorrhage. Other series have demonstrated that infarcts can be seen, can be hyperechoic acutely, and become isoechoic with time, or present as hypoechoic lesions. Placental infarcts typically occur along the *maternal* plate of the placenta (see Fig. A).

The differential diagnosis of larger infarcts includes hemorrhage or hematoma, which will decrease in size and change in appearance with time. Three additional focal placental abnormalities include fibrin deposition, chorioangioma and intervillous thrombosis. Fibrin deposition is more common on the *fetal* side of the placenta. Chorioangiomas are vascular masses of mixed echogenicity that usually present in the first half of the gestation. Later in gestation, an intervillous thrombosis may be detected as a hypoechoic region with slow, turbulent flow.

Notes

Papillary Muscle Calcification (Intraventricular Hyperechoic Focus)

1. Papillary muscle calcification.

2. Histologic studies show an incidence of 17%.

3. Calcification in a papillary muscle.

4. No, except if bilateral.

References

Manning JE, Ragavendra N, Sayre J, et al: Significance of fetal intracardiac echogenic foci in relation to trisomy 21: A prospective sonographic study of high-risk pregnant women. *AJR Am J Roentgenol* 170:1083–1084, 1998.

Wax JR, Philput C: Fetal intracardiac echogenic foci: Does it matter which ventricle? *J Ultrasound Med* 17:141–144, 1998.

Cross-Reference

Ultrasound: THE REQUISITES, p 242.

Comment

The intracardiac hyperechoic focus is a 1- to 2-mm punctate bright reflector within a papillary muscle. It is found most commonly in the left ventricle but can arise in the right ventricle or can be biventricular. Biventricular calcification is more frequently associated with aneuploidy. Isolated right or left ventricular calcification is often an isolated finding, without significance but may occasionally be associated with structural anomalies.

Pathologically, the focus represents papillary muscle microcalcification. Histologic studies have shown that this calcification is present in 15% to 17% of aneuploid fetuses versus 2% to 5% of normals. The significance of this finding is controversial when seen on an ultrasound examination. In a *high-risk* population, a statistically significant association has been shown with Down syndrome (trisomy 21). Because this finding is present in only 13% of fetuses with Down syndrome, compared with 2% of normal fetuses, the positive predictive value is low. Many other studies have shown no increased incidence of Down syndrome in fetuses with the intracardiac hyperechoic focus. At present, the incidence of gross calcifications detected by ultrasound probably increases the risk of Down syndrome by no more than a factor of 2.

Detection of this as an isolated finding in the general population necessitates at most an echocardiographic examination for structural anomalies. In a high-risk population (e.g., advanced maternal age, abnormal triple screen), an additional careful evaluation for other systemic malformations is warranted.

Notes

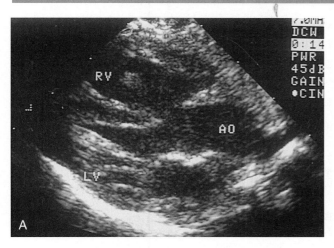

1. What abnormalities are demonstrated on this outflow view of a third-trimester fetal heart (Fig. A. RV = right ventricle; LV = left ventricle; AO = aorta)?

2. What is the most likely cause?

3. How do the ventricles appear on a four-chamber view in tetralogy of Fallot?

4. What is the differential diagnosis of aortic enlargement with a small pulmonary artery?

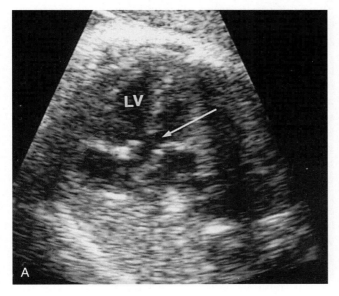 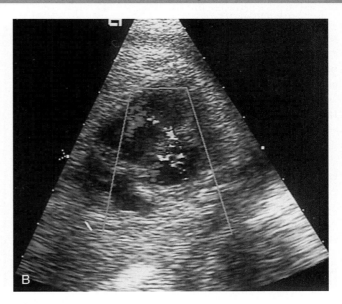

1. What is the defect (arrow) shown on this four-chamber view of a mid–second-trimester fetal heart (Figs. A and B)? Figure B is a color Doppler image in different orientation compared with Figure A.

2. What are the four types?

3. What fetal echocardiographic view best demonstrates this anomaly?

4. What is the effect on fetal cardiac hemodynamics?

Tetralogy of Fallot

1. Ventricular septal defect (VSD) and an enlarged overriding aorta.

2. Tetralogy of Fallot.

3. Most commonly normal.

4. Tetralogy of Fallot and a hypoplastic right heart.

Acknowledgment

Figure for Case 39 courtesy of Mr. Dennis Wood.

References

Benacerraf BR: Sonographic detection of fetal anomalies of the aortic and pulmonary arteries: Value of the four-chamber view vs. direct images. *AJR Am J Roentgenol* 163:1483–1489, 1994.

Brown DL, DiSalvo DN, Frates MC, et al: Sonography of the fetal heart: Normal variants and pitfalls. *AJR Am J Roentgenol* 160:1251–1255, 1993.

Cross-Reference

Ultrasound: THE REQUISITES, pp 238–243.

Comment

Tetralogy of Fallot is one of the more common complex cardiac malformations and includes a VSD with overriding aorta, pulmonic stenosis, and right ventricular infundibular obstruction. There are variable degrees of pulmonary artery atresia. Tetralogy of Fallot can be seen in various syndromes, including Down syndrome. In addition the branchial arch defects are associated (DiGeorge syndrome, velocardiofacial syndrome, and conotruncal anomaly face syndrome). Almost 40% of patients with tetralogy of Fallot have additional cardiac anomalies, particularly if tetralogy of Fallot is associated with one of these syndromes. In addition, all patients with tetralogy of Fallot have an increased incidence of noncardiac as well as chromosomal anomalies.

On prenatal sonogram, the four-chamber view is most commonly normal, with symmetric ventricular size. However, outflow views reveal a large overriding aorta and a VSD (see Fig. A). It is important to recognize that one can create a "pseudo-overriding aorta" on the long axis view of the left ventricular outflow tract. If the aorta is truly overriding in the setting of tetralogy of Fallot, the vessel should be enlarged and the abnormality will persist despite the orientation of scanning. The pseudo-overriding aorta may be due to volume averaging with the pulmonary artery or sinus of Valsalva.

Tetralogy of Fallot is the most common anomaly with a discrepancy in the size of the aorta to pulmonary outflow tract. The differential diagnosis includes hypoplastic right heart.

Notes

Ventriculoseptal Defect

1. Ventriculoseptal defect (VSD).

2. Perimembranous, muscular, supracristal, and atrioventricular (AV) canal.

3. The four-chamber view.

4. Usually has no effect on *fetal* cardiac hemodynamics.

Acknowledgment

Figures for Case 40 courtesy of Mr. Dennis Wood.

References

Nacht A, Kronzon I: Intracardiac shunts. *Crit Care Clin* 12:295–319, 1996.

Soto B, Bargeron LM, Diethelm E: Ventricular septal defect. *Semin Roentgenol* 10:200–213, 1985.

Cross-Reference

Ultrasound: THE REQUISITES, pp 237–243.

Comment

A VSD is the most common isolated congenital cardiac defect. In addition, it is present in conjunction with numerous other cardiac malformations, including tetralogy of Fallot, transposition of the great vessels, pulmonic atresia, and double-outlet right ventricle.

There are four types of VSDs, depending on their location. The most common type involves the lower membranous septum. The second type occurs in the muscular septum and can have multiple defects. Trisomy 21 is associated with the third type, an AV canal. In these cases, atrial and ventricular defects are present with anomalous AV valves. The last type is the supracristal defect, which is located directly below the aortic valve and is associated with aortic insufficiency.

Prenatal diagnosis of low membranous and muscular defects relies on an adequate four-chamber view of the heart and outlet views. Whereas the four-chamber view detects approximately 50% of cases, the sensitivity is approximately 80% when outlet views are incorporated. Ultrasound can demonstrate an interruption in the ventricular septum (see Fig. A). It is essential to image the septum perpendicular to the beam of the ultrasound transducer to avoid a pseudo-defect caused by dropout. This case demonstrates the utility of color Doppler to depict the flow between the ventricles (see Fig. B). Small defects can be missed, and high defects require views to image the subaortic region. Once diagnosed, a careful search should be conducted for other cardiac anomalies, which are present in 40% of cases, using longitudinal and short axis views of the great vessels.

Notes

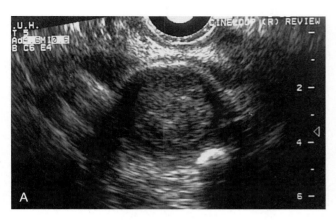

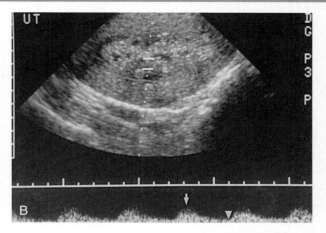

1. In this 70-year-old woman who presents with vaginal bleeding, what is the primary finding and what is the most likely diagnosis (Fig. A)? Figure A shows an axial/coronal transvaginal examination of the uterus.

2. Does spectral Doppler imaging in another postmenopausal patient confirm the diagnosis (Fig. B)? Figure B is a split image. The upper half shows a sagittal transvaginal study of the uterus with the Doppler cursor on the thickened endometrium. The lower half shows an arterial waveform; peak systole is noted by arrow and end-diastole is marked by an arrowhead.

3. What is an important question to ask the patient with a thickened endometrium?

4. Is endometrial hyperplasia considered to be premalignant?

C A S E   4 2

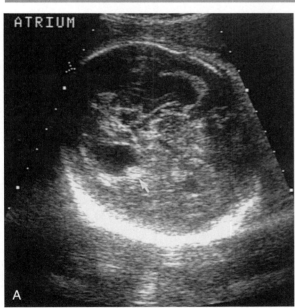

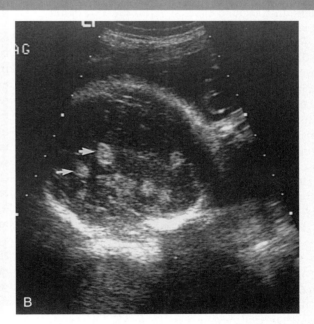

1. In the mid–second-trimester ultrasound, the fetal head is small. In transaxial and oblique views, what are the most likely causes of the hyperechoic areas denoted by arrows and what is the most likely diagnosis (Figs. A and B)?

2. What is the most common in utero infection in the United States?

3. What are the central nervous system (CNS) findings in the fetus with a TORCH (*t*oxoplasmosis, *o*ther infections, *r*ubella, *c*ytomegalovirus (CMV), *h*erpes/human immunodeficiency virus [HIV]) infection?

4. What is the prognosis for the fetus?

Endometrial Cancer

1. Marked heterogeneous endometrial thickening. Endometrial cancer.

2. Yes. High diastolic flow suggests a malignancy.

3. For a premenopausal woman, "When was the last menstrual period?" For a postmenopausal woman, "Are you taking hormonal replacement supplements?"

4. Yes, the atypical subtype.

References

Karlsson B, Granberg S, Wikland M: Transvaginal ultrasonography of the endometrium in women with postmenopausal bleeding—a Nordic multicenter study. *Am J Obstet Gynecol* 173:1637–1638, 1995.

Kurjak A, Shalan J, Sosic A, et al: Endometrial carcinoma in postmenopausal women: Evaluation by transvaginal color Doppler ultrasonography. *Am J Obstet Gynecol* 169:1597–1602, 1993.

Cross-Reference

Ultrasound: THE REQUISITES, pp 368–374.

Comment

Endometrial cancer usually occurs in women older than 50 years of age, most of whom present with postmenopausal bleeding. These cases of endometrial cancer demonstrate that the neoplasm often causes greater degrees of endometrial thickening than other benign etiologies (see Figs. A and B). One series using transvaginal ultrasound demonstrated that the endometrium in endometrial cancer was almost always greater than 10 mm (90% of cases) and usually greater than 20 mm in thickness. The thickened endometrium is usually hyperechoic or heterogeneous and is rarely hypoechoic. Vascularity can be seen in or around the tumor in most cases; the arterial flow often demonstrates a low resistive index (<0.4) and elevated peak systolic velocity (see Fig. B). Color Doppler sonography can confirm myometrial invasion by detecting an interruption of the zone of decreased echogenicity in the subendometrial region.

Thickening of the endometrium is the first indicator on ultrasound that an endometrial abnormality is present. In young women, the normal endometrium can measure up to 15 mm, depending on the phase of their menstrual cycle. On a sonohysterogram, the single-layer thickness of the endometrium should be normally less than 3 mm. Postmenopausal women should have a double-layer thickness less than 5 mm. Patients on tamoxifen therapy and women taking hormone supplements postmenopausally are allowed a normal thickness up to 8 mm.

Notes

In Utero Infection

1. Arrows = parenchymal calcifications. Cytomegalovirus (CMV).

2. CMV.

3. Microcephaly, periventricular calcifications, hydrocephalus, cerebellar aplasia, encephalomalacia, and porencephaly.

4. The prognosis is poor.

Reference

Drose JA, Dennis MA, Thickman D: Infection in utero: US findings in 19 cases. *Radiology* 178:369–374, 1991.

Cross-Reference

Ultrasound: THE REQUISITES, pp 214–215.

Comment

In utero infection in the United States is most often caused by cytomegalovirus. Other infectious agents include varicella, syphilis, herpes simplex type 2, listeriosis, and toxoplasmosis as well as HIV. Death can occur in utero or in the neonatal period, and those that survive may have developmental impairment or mental retardation.

The infection is often subclinical in the mother and is detected by the development of serum antibodies or isolating the virus from urine or the cervix. Alternatively, amniocentesis or cordocentesis will document exposure of the fetus to the infection, although it does not predict the impact on fetal development.

Anomalies can occur in various organs. CNS malformations include hydrocephalus, microcephaly, cerebellar aplasia, encephalomalacia, or porencephaly. Ultrasound may demonstrate periventricular and parenchymal calcifications (see Figs. A and B). Much less commonly, the tubers of tuberous sclerosis may present in a microcephalic fetus as hyperechoic intracranial masses.

Cardiac anomalies include septal defects, cardiomegaly, and pulmonary stenosis. Hepatosplenomegaly, pleural effusion, ascites, and hydrops may be identified as well as intra-abdominal (including hepatic) calcifications. The amount of amniotic fluid can vary from oligohydramnios to polyhydramnios. Intrauterine growth restriction develops in some cases. The placenta was enlarged in 30% of one series. In some cases, the abnormalities may not be present on the first ultrasound but may develop later in the gestation. In any prenatal sonogram in which unusual or atypical anomalies are detected, in utero infection should be considered.

Notes

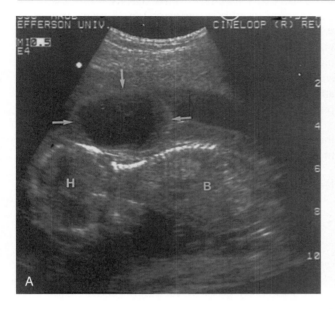

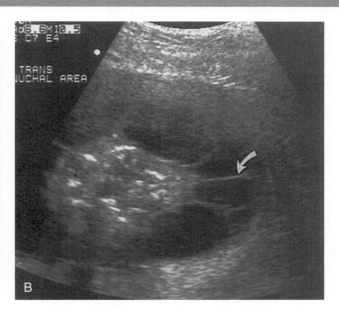

1. What is the abnormality located posterior to the fetal neck, and what is the most common chromosomal abnormality associated with it (Fig. A is sagittal. H = head; B = body)? Figure B is an axial view of the neck. Is there an association with any other aneuploid states?

2. What percentage of pregnancies with this anomaly results in a healthy neonate with a normal karyotype?

3. What structure accounts for the midline septum (see Fig. B, curved arrow) in this cystic lesion?

4. What additional diffuse fetal findings may be associated?

C A S E   4 3

Cystic Hygroma

1. Cystic hygroma. Turner's syndrome (XO). Yes, also with trisomy 21, 18, and 13 and others.

2. Very few—only 9%.

3. Nuchal ligament or septation.

4. Nonimmune hydrops. (Fig. C, axial image of the abdomen [L = liver])

Reference
Descamps P, Jourdain O, Paillet C, et al: Etiology, prognosis and management of nuchal cystic hygroma: 25 new cases and literature review. *Eur J Obstet Gynecol Reprod Biol* 71:3–10, 1997.

Cross-Reference
Ultrasound: THE REQUISITES, pp 232–234.

Comment
Cystic hygroma (see Figs. A and B) is a multiloculated septated cystic neck mass comprised of dilated lymphatics. It is most commonly associated with Turner's syndrome, but other chromosomal anomalies associated include trisomies 13, 18, and 21 as well as more rare mendelian chromosomal abnormalities. Only 9% of neonates born with this anomaly will be healthy with normal chromosomes. Associated nonchromosomal abnormalities include Noonan's syndrome, multiple pterygium disease, Cowchock's syndrome, and Robert's syndrome as well as chondrodystrophies.

The α-fetoprotein (AFP) level varies, ranging from normal to very high. Lymphedema is present in slightly more than 50% of cases. Nonimmune hydrops is a complication that carries almost 100% mortality, owing to a diffuse lymphatic obstruction (see Fig. C); the risk correlates with the size of the hygroma. Oligohydramnios is commonly present.

Cystic hygroma may resolve in utero; nonetheless, karyotyping should be performed in all cases. In fetuses with a normal karyotype, parental karyotyping is advised to predict the risk of a recurrence. If parents have a normal karyotype, there is no increased risk in subsequent pregnancies. Cases that appear late (usually anterior or lateral in the neck) may have a different pathophysiology with a better prognosis.

The differential diagnosis of a posterior cystic neck mass includes an occipital encephalocele and a cervical myelomeningocele.

Notes

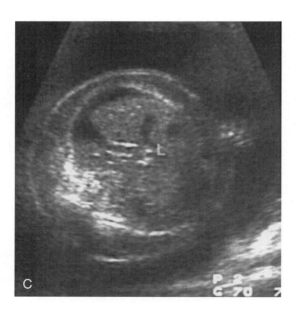

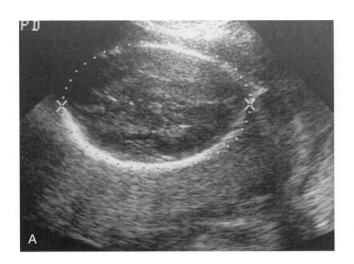

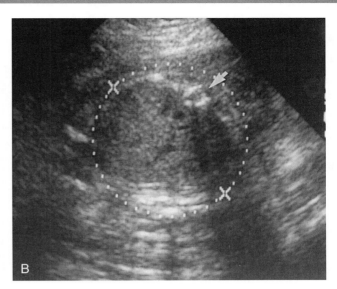

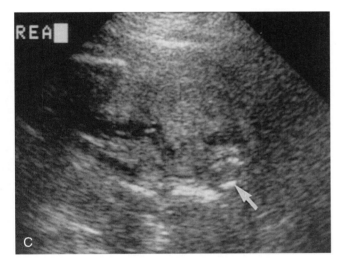

1. What are the findings identified in this second-trimester fetus (Figs. A to C), and what is the most likely diagnosis? Figure A is an axial image of the fetal head. Figure B is an axial image of the upper fetal abdomen, and Figure C is an axial image of the renal areas. (Arrow = spine.)

2. What quantitative measure is used to evaluate the severity of decreased amniotic fluid?

3. What clinical symptom(s) might the mother report in the setting of severe oligohydramnios?

4. What additional evaluation should be performed once this finding is made?

C A S E 4 4

Oligohydramnios (Secondary to Renal Agenesis)

1. Severe oligohydramnios and absence of the kidneys. The most likely diagnosis is bilateral renal agenesis.

2. Measuring an amniotic fluid index (AFI).

3. Decreased fetal movement, leaking amniotic fluid.

4. Umbilical artery Doppler.

References

Cunningham FG, MacDonald PC, Gant NF, et al: *Williams Obstetrics,* 20th ed. Stamford, CT, Appleton & Lange, 1997, pp 664–665.

Sepulveda W, Stagiannis KD, Flack NJ, Fisk NM: Accuracy of prenatal diagnosis of renal agenesis with color flow imaging in severe second-trimester oligohydramnios. *Am J Obstet Gynecol* 173:1788–1792, 1995.

Cross-Reference

Ultrasound: THE REQUISITES, pp 276–277.

Comment

Abnormalities in amniotic fluid volume reflect underlying fetal, maternal, and placental conditions. Oligohydramnios is defined as fluid volume less than the fifth percentile for a specific gestational age. The amniotic fluid volume varies with the gestational age and peaks in the second trimester. Although the diagnosis can be made by measuring the fluid (usually in the four uterine quadrants) as four perpendicular measurements added together, a subjective evaluation of the amount of fluid is usually equally or more precise.

As this case of bilateral renal agenesis demonstrates, the abnormality in amniotic fluid volume may be immediately apparent (see Figs. A to C). Severe oligohydramnios should prompt a directed scan to identify the cause. The anatomy should be evaluated for the presence of both kidneys (see Fig. C) and fluid in the urinary bladder, both of which are absent in bilateral renal agenesis. The adrenal glands are large in utero and can resemble the kidneys; the urinary bladder will still not be present. A severe bilateral renal obstruction or any other bilateral renal anomaly that affects function (i.e., a multicystic dysplastic kidney with a contralateral ureteropelvic junction obstruction) would also lead to severe oligohydramnios.

If the fluid volume is very low, the anatomy can be difficult to assess. Color Doppler has been shown to be useful in documenting the presence of renal arteries to exclude renal agenesis in these cases.

Alternative causes of oligohydramnios include growth restriction (intrauterine growth restriction or intrauterine growth retardation), chromosomal anomalies, some congenital anomalies (e.g., cystic hygroma), and fetal demise. Hypertension, diabetes, and preeclampsia are among the maternal causes. Placental insufficiency, a cause of oligohydramnios later in the gestation, warrants umbilical artery Doppler imaging whenever the fluid volume appears low. To exclude rupture of the membranes as the cause, the mother should be asked about any symptoms of fluid leakage. A physical examination must be conducted immediately by the obstetrician to exclude ruptured membranes, and the examination should be performed using a sterile speculum and the "fern test."

Notes

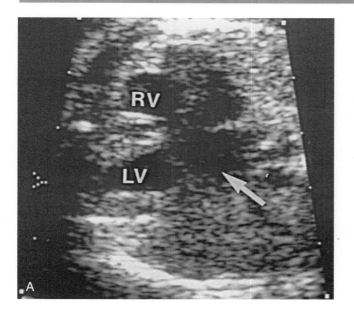

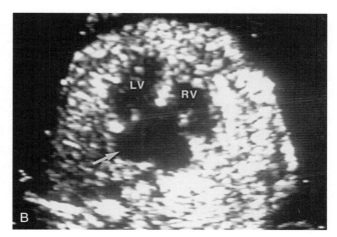

1. What is the anomaly shown in the four-chamber cardiac images of two second-trimester fetuses (Figs. A and B. LV = left ventricle; RV = right ventricle; arrow = left atrium)? What chromosomal anomaly is associated with this cardiac malformation?

2. What other cardiac malformations are associated with this cardiac malformation?

3. What subtype of this cardiac anomaly includes obstructive lesions of the right or left ventricle?

4. What percentage have significant atrioventricular (AV) valve regurgitation?

Endocardial Cushion Defect

1. Endocardial cushion AV canal defects. Down syndrome (70%).

2. Tetralogy of Fallot (10%).

3. Unbalanced AV canal.

4. 20%.

Acknowledgment

Figures for Case 45 courtesy of Mr. Dennis Wood.

Reference

Pearl JM, Laks H: Intermediate and complete forms of atrioventricular canal. *Semin Thorac Cardiovasc Surg* 9:8–20, 1997.

Cross-Reference

Ultrasound: THE REQUISITES, pp 238–243.

Comment

The AV canal, or endocardial cushion defect, is a cardiac malformation defined by a common AV valve with superior and inferior bridging leaflets that divide an otherwise continuous septal defect of atria and ventricles. Both of these cases demonstrate the AV septal defect. A classification system was described by Rastelli (types A to C), depending on the morphology of the superior bridging valve leaflet.

Ten percent of patients with AV canal also have tetralogy of Fallot. A complete endocardial cushion defect is associated with Down syndrome in 70% of cases and is the most common congenital cardiac malformation in Down syndrome. In non–Down syndrome cases, there is an increased incidence of an "unbalanced AV canal," where an obstructive lesion or hypoplasia of one of the ventricles is also present and dictates a different type of surgical repair.

A four-chamber view of the fetal heart easily identifies this abnormality by the mid-second trimester. Whereas ventricular and atrial septal defects by themselves could be small and missed, the combined defect forming an AV canal (see Figs. A and B) is accurately diagnosed. Accompanying arrhythmias may also be detected.

Treatment at the present time usually entails complete surgical repair in infancy. The older treatment of preliminary pulmonary banding is now reserved for infants who are not good surgical candidates, either due to sepsis, congestive heart failure, organ dysfunction, associated malformations, or small infants whose anatomy is difficult to correct surgically. The long-term outcome appears to be worse for those with Down syndrome and is attributed to the degree of pulmonary vascular disease in these patients.

Notes

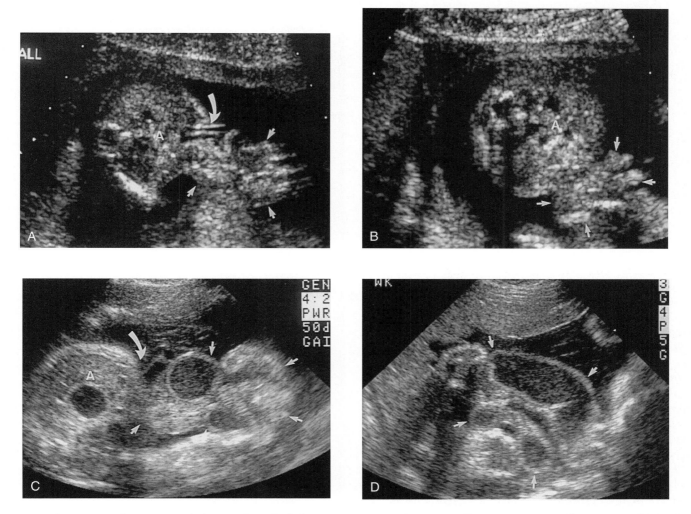

1. What type of anterior abdominal wall defect (arrows) is shown in these two second-trimester fetuses (fetus 1, Figs. A and B; fetus 2, Figs. C and D)? A = fetal abdomen. What does the curved arrow in Figures A and C represent?

2. How is gastroschisis distinguished from an omphalocele with prenatal ultrasound?

3. What prenatal ultrasound finding carries a higher incidence of postnatal bowel complication in gastroschisis?

4. Are there any associated anomalies?

Gastroschisis

1. Gastroschisis. Curved arrow = a normal umbilical cord insertion.

2. Paraumbilical location of the defect, and the lack of a covering peritoneal membrane.

3. Small bowel diameter greater than 11 mm.

4. Only secondary gastrointestinal abnormalities. This literature does not consistently report increased incidence of other anomalies.

References

Babcook CH, Hedrick MH, Goldstein RB, et al: Gastroschisis: Can sonography of the fetal bowel accurately predict postnatal outcome? *J Ultrasound Med* 13:701–706, 1994.

Emanuel PG, Garcia GI, Angtuaco TL: Prenatal detection of anterior abdominal wall defects with ultrasound. *Radiographics* 15:517–530, 1995.

Cross-Reference

Ultrasound: THE REQUISITES, pp 268–269.

Comment

Gastroschisis is an isolated, eccentrically placed, anterior abdominal wall defect. As opposed to an omphalocele, the abdominal wall defect in gastroschisis is paraumbilical, usually on the right side in the lower quadrant (see Figs. A and C), but occasionally it is found in the left lower quadrant. The anterior abdominal wall defect is believed to be caused by ischemia secondary to disruption of the omphalomesenteric artery or a weakening in the anterior abdominal wall secondary to right umbilical vein involution.

Bowel herniates through the defect with no overlying membrane, accounting for the absence of fetal ascites, and the much higher maternal serum AFP levels compared with an omphalocele.

Gastrointestinal abnormalities can result, including malrotation, bowel atresia, or stenosis. It is important to evaluate the caliber of the bowel, because dilatation indicates an increased incidence of postnatal bowel complications (fetus 2, see Figs. C and D). A study by Babcook and associates demonstrated that on prenatal ultrasound, a maximum small bowel diameter of greater than 11 mm was seen more frequently in fetuses that had complications such as obstruction or atresia, necrosis, or the need for postnatal bowel resection. Others have believed that the bowel caliber has to be greater (as large as 17 mm in diameter) before these complications occur universally. Meconium peritonitis is suggested by dilatation and wall thickening of bowel within the abdomen (see Fig. C, a cystic structure adjacent to the letter A).

Most of the literature reports no increased incidence in other anomalies compared with normal patients. Accordingly, the prognosis is better than that with an omphalocele. The condition of the bowel at the time of delivery dictates the postnatal prognosis. Ischemic bowel, sepsis, and premature delivery are leading causes of death.

Notes

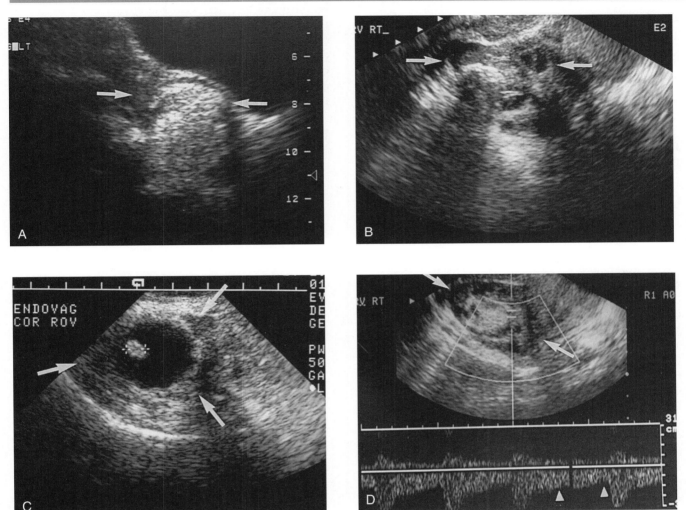

1. Four women, who are 20 to 35 years of age, present with ovarian masses (Figs. A to D, denoted by arrows). Figure A is a transabominal sagittal image of the left ovary. Figure B is a transvaginal axial/coronal image of the right ovary. Figure C is a transvaginal coronal image of the right ovary. Figure D is a split image, with the upper half showing a transvaginal axial/coronal image of the right ovary and the lower half showing a spectral Doppler waveform. What is the most likely common diagnosis in these cases?

2. What are three complications associated with this mass?

3. What structure(s) account for the "bright lines and dots" often seen in these masses with sonography?

4. What endocrine syndrome is rarely associated and why?

Dermoid

1. Dermoid (cystic teratoma).

2. Torsion, infection, and rare malignant degeneration.

3. Hair.

4. Thyrotoxicosis; the presence of struma ovarii in the tumor.

References

Patel MD, Feldstein VA, Lipson SD, et al: Cystic teratomas of the ovary: Diagnostic value of sonography. *AJR Am J Roentgenol* 171:1061–1065, 1998.

Zalel Y, Caspi B, Tepper R: Doppler flow characteristics of dermoid cysts: Unique appearance of struma ovarii. *J Ultrasound Med* 16:355–358, 1997.

Cross-Reference

Ultrasound: THE REQUISITES, pp 400–403.

Comment

Mature cystic teratomas, also known as dermoid cysts, are the most common ovarian tumors, comprising up to 25% of all ovarian neoplasms. They are often incidental findings on cross-sectional imaging and can be bilateral in a few cases. However, because they are very mobile, they can be difficult to detect on bimanual pelvic examination and can, especially if large, cause ovarian torsion. Other complications include infection and rare malignant degeneration. Once discovered, management is usually by surgical excision to prevent the known complications. If the dermoid is small, it may be removed without loss of the entire ovary.

The ultrasound appearance depends on which components are present (see Figs. A to D). Mature *dermoids* arise from ectoderm; mature *teratomas* consist of any of the three mature germ cell layers: ectoderm, mesoderm, and endoderm. Macroscopically, they contain variable amounts of sebum, hair, and teeth. The dermoid plug, or Rokitansky protuberance, consists of sebaceous material as well as calcifications or teeth (see Fig. B), hair, and other soft tissue; this dermoid plug is present in most teratomas and varies in size. It is seen on ultrasound as a hyperechoic nodule or mass with shadowing, often within a more simple appearing cyst (see Fig. C; +'s denote hyperechoic nodule). The cyst is filled with homogeneous sebaceous fluid, which accounts for the lack of internal echoes. Several characteristic ultrasound findings have been described for dermoids. Diffuse or regional bright echoes may be seen (see Figs. A and D). As in Figure A, the echogenicity is brightest at the top, with absorption of sound internally, called the "tip of the iceberg" sign. The presence of hair accounts for hyperechoic lines and dots (see Fig. A). A fluid-fluid level can be present.

In up to 20% of cases, thyroid tissue is present microscopically. When thyroid tissue constitutes a large portion of the lesion, it is called struma ovarii. In these cases, women may present with thyrotoxicosis or thyroid enlargement. On ultrasound, if the mass is endocrine secreting, a solid component will be seen in the dermoid with low impedance arterial flow detected by Doppler ultrasound (see Fig. D, arrowheads).

Notes

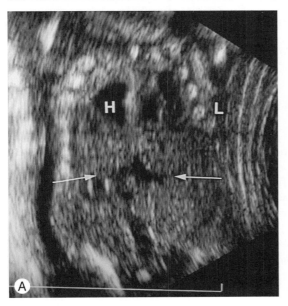

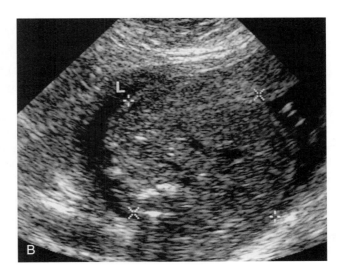

1. What is the diagnosis in this second-trimester fetus? Figure A is a coronal image of the fetal chest and abdomen (arrows = the diaphragm; H = the heart; L = left side of the fetus). Figure B is an axial image of the upper fetal abdomen (L = left side of the fetus).
2. Are there associated anomalies?
3. What prenatal measurements help to predict survival?
4. What finding aids in distinguishing congenital diaphragmatic hernia (CDH) from cystic adenomatoid malformation (CAM)?

C A S E   4 9

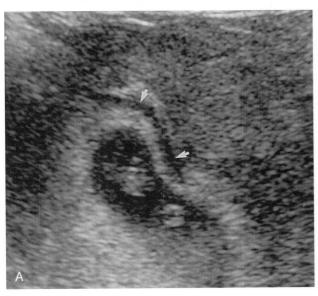

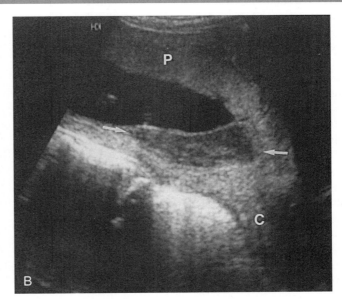

1. Figure A is a first-trimester scan of a gestational sac. Figure B is a sagittal image of a third-trimester pregnancy (P = placenta; C = cervix). What is the finding shown by arrows, and what is the usual presentation of these pregnant women?
2. What is the overall spontaneous abortion rate if this abnormality is present?
3. What is the spontaneous abortion rate in normal (uncomplicated) pregnancies with a living fetus seen by ultrasound at less than 12 weeks?
4. What three factors influence the outcome in cases such as the one shown here?

C A S E 4 8

Congenital Diaphragmatic Hernia, Left-Sided Bochdalek

1. Left-sided diaphragmatic hernia (Bochdalek).

2. Yes.

3. Quantification of the contralateral lung area and an assessment of ventricular symmetry.

4. Paucity of abdominal contents.

References

Guibaud L, Filiatrault D, Garel L, et al: Fetal congenital diaphragmatic hernia: Accuracy of sonography in the diagnosis and prediction of the outcome after birth. *AJR Am J Roentgenol* 166:1195–1202, 1996.

Hubard AM, Adzick NS, Crombleholme TM, Haselgrove JC: Left-sided congenital diaphragmatic hernia: Value of prenatal MR imaging in preparation for fetal surgery. *Radiology* 203:636–640, 1997.

Cross-Reference
Ultrasound: THE REQUISITES, pp 245–246.

Comment

CDH can occur laterally (Bochdalek) or medially (Morgagni). Abdominal contents (e.g., stomach, bowel, liver, mesenteric fat) can herniate into the thorax. Pulmonary hypoplasia and pulmonary hypertension result from compression of the ipsilateral and contralateral lung. Associated malformations include congenital heart disease and chromosomal anomalies.

Left-sided Bochdalek hernias, as shown in this case, are much more common. Ultrasound reveals cystic and solid structures in the left hemithorax. Coronal views (see Fig. A) are particularly useful for demonstrating a supradiaphragmatic stomach or bowel. If herniated, the stomach will not be identified in the abdomen on a standard axial view (see Fig. B). Shift of the heart and mediastinum are common. Polyhydramnios is associated and has a worse prognosis if it occurs early in the gestation. Herniation of the left lobe of the liver carries a poor prognosis because of difficulty in postnatal surgical repair. It may be difficult to distinguish hyperechoic herniated contents from the ipsilateral lung.

The contralateral residual lung area has been shown to correlate with the outcome. If the contralateral lung area is equal to or greater than half of the hemithorax, the survival rate is often higher. Another assessment of the contralateral lung volume is the ratio of contralateral lung to head circumference. Disproportion of the cardiac ventricles is a predictor of a poor outcome.

Notes

C A S E 4 9

Subchorionic Hemorrhage

1. Hemorrhage. Vaginal bleeding.

2. 9%.

3. 2%.

4. Hemorrhage volume, gestational age, and maternal age.

Reference

Bennet GL, Bromley B, Lieberman E, Benacerraf BR: Subchorionic hemorrhage in the first-trimester pregnancies: Prediction of pregnancy outcome with sonography. *Radiology* 200:803–806, 1996.

Cross-Reference
Ultrasound: THE REQUISITES, pp 317–327.

Comment

The differential diagnosis of a pregnant woman who presents with vaginal bleeding in the first trimester includes spontaneous abortion (miscarriage), ectopic pregnancy, anembryonic pregnancy, molar pregnancy, and subchorionic hemorrhage.

Early in the gestation, a hemorrhage is often within the endometrial canal but may be subchorionic. Later in the pregnancy, if the hemorrhage has not decompressed by vaginal bleeding, it is often identified below the amniochorionic membrane (either subchorionic if over the placenta or submembranous if anywhere else). On ultrasound, a first-trimester hemorrhage appears as a crescentic or oval-shaped fluid collection adjacent to the gestational sac in the endometrial canal (see Fig. A, arrows). It is important not to confuse an unfused amniotic membrane (chorionic-amniotic separation), a normal finding that may be seen up to 16 weeks. In the second and third trimesters, a hemorrhage appears as a crescentic or ovoid-shaped mass projecting into the amniotic space (see Fig. B, arrows).

The echogenicity varies with the age of the hemorrhage. The bleed is anechoic acutely, becomes heterogeneous in the subacute stage, and eventually resumes an anechoic appearance when chronic. Follow-up studies are imperative to confirm a decrease in size and progressive liquification (becoming anechoic).

Studies have shown that the spontaneous abortion rate is increased in these patients from a baseline of 2% to 9% when a subchorionic hemorrhage is identified early in the gestation. The outcome depends on the size of the hemorrhage (volume), the gestational age of the fetus, and the maternal age. The prognosis is worse for larger hemorrhages, fetuses of 8 weeks' gestational age or younger, and women 35 years of age or older.

Notes

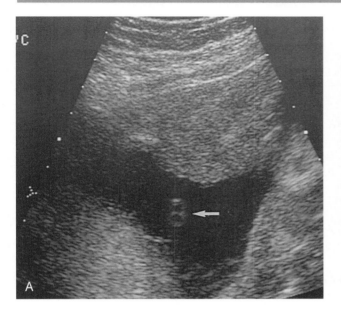

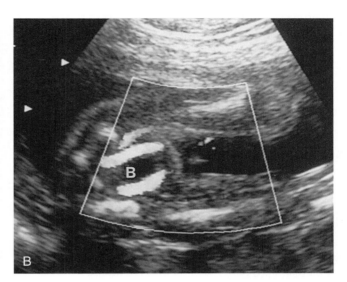

1. In Figure A, what is the finding in this cross-sectional image of the umbilical cord (arrow)? What is its clinical significance when the fetus has no other anomaly?
2. What central nervous system (CNS) anomalies have been associated?
3. What is the most common associated chromosomal anomaly?
4. What is shown by this color Doppler axial image of the fetal pelvis of another fetus (Fig. B; B = urinary bladder)?

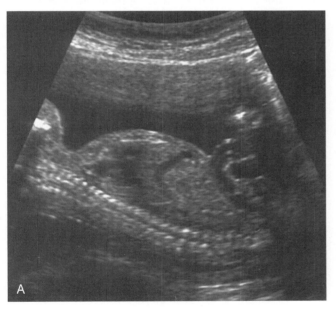

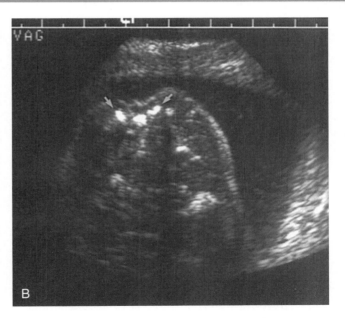

1. What does the transvaginal scan (Fig. B, axial view of lower lumbar spine) demonstrate in this case that was not apparent on the initial transabdominal image (Fig. A, sagittal image of fetus in breech position) and why?
2. What percentage of these fetuses with this disorder have a karyotype abnormality?
3. Other than gestational age, what factor correlates with the degree of ventriculomegaly in these fetuses?
4. Where is α-fetoprotein (AFP) produced, and when does fetal serum AFP peak?

C A S E 5 0

Single Umbilical Artery (Two-Vessel Umbilical Cord)

1. Two-vessel umbilical cord. In the absence of fetal malformations, there is no clinical significance.

2. Holoprosencephaly, hydrocephalus, and cerebellar dysgenesis.

3. Trisomy 18.

4. Bilateral internal iliac arteries.

References
Dudiak CM, Salomon CG, Posniak HV, et al: Sonography of the umbilical cord. *Radiographics* 15:1035–1050, 1995.

Nyberg DA, Mahony BS, Luthy D, Kapur R: Single umbilical artery: Prenatal detection of concurrent anomalies. *J Ultrasound Med* 10:247–253, 1991.

Cross-Reference
Ultrasound: THE REQUISITES, pp 313–315.

Comment
The presence of a single umbilical artery (a two-vessel umbilical cord) is a marker for concurrent fetal anomalies in 20% to 50% of singleton gestations where it is detected. Ultrasound reveals two vessels on cross-sectional imaging of the cord: a single umbilical artery, which may be as large as the adjacent umbilical vein (see Fig. A). When a two-vessel umbilical cord is suspected, however, care must be taken to evaluate the entire cord, especially close to the fetal insertion. In the development of the cord, part of it may be two vessels and part may consist of three vessels. If three vessels are detected in any part, more commonly occurring closer to the fetus, then the cord is considered to have three vessels. Color Doppler imaging of the fetal pelvis can often help to confirm the presence or absence of two internal iliac arteries (one on each side of the bladder [Fig. B]) supplying the two umbilical arteries.

The importance of the ultrasound examination is to exclude additional anomalies. Marginal and velamentous cord insertions have been associated. Interestingly, the infants with a single umbilical artery and no other congenital or chromosomal anomaly have an increased risk of an inguinal hernia.

CNS associated anomalies include holoprosencephaly, hydrocephalus, and cerebellar dysgenesis. Various complex cardiac malformations, gastrointestinal abnormalities (omphalocele and congenital diaphragmatic hernia), musculoskeletal and genitourinary anomalies have also been described. Trisomy 18 is the most common chromosomal anomaly; trisomy 13, Turner's syndrome, and triploidy are also associated.

Notes

C A S E 5 1

Myelomeningocele

1. Spinal dysraphism due to a myelomeningocele; the spine is not adequately evaluated in Figure A.

2. 13% to 17%.

3. The severity of the posterior fossa defect.

4. Fetal liver and yolk sac; 12 to 13 weeks' gestation.

Reference
Babcook CJ, Goldstein RV, Filly RA: Prenatally detected fetal myelomeningocele: Is karyotype analysis warranted? *Radiology* 194:491-494, 1995.

Cross-Reference
Ultrasound: THE REQUISITES, pp 228–232.

Comment
Imaging of the entire fetal spine is essential, especially the lumbosacral region. In this case, the fetus was in a relatively poor position for complete evaluation—breech presentation with the spine down (see Fig. A). The lumbosacral region could at best be only partially imaged. Because the lower spine was close to the lower uterine segment, a transvaginal examination that is usually limited to first-trimester evaluation allowed complete visualization of the lumbosacral spine and in a better plane or section (see Fig. B). The posterior elements are abnormally splayed outward (arrows), and the overlying posterior soft tissues are absent.

A careful survey of the fetal spine is essential with prenatal ultrasound. Each vertebral body should have three ossification centers. The two posterior ossification centers must be parallel or converge. Divergence can be detected in axial and coronal planes in a myelomeningocele. A fluid-filled mass is usually seen overlying the defect. Associated musculoskeletal findings include clubfoot and scoliosis or kyphosis. Movement of the lower extremities of the fetus does not correlate with postnatal motor function.

Karyotype abnormalities occur in 13% to 17% of fetuses with spina bifida. In 20% of these cases, a prenatal sonogram shows only spina bifida. The presence of an NTD should prompt a careful search for other anomalies which, if present, significantly raise the likelihood of a karyotype abnormality.

Notes

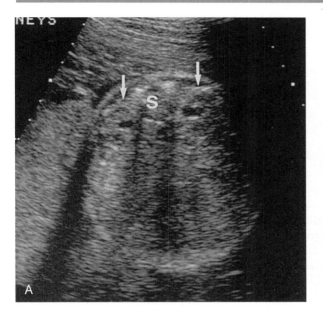

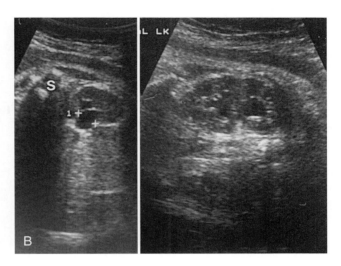

1. Is there an abnormality in either of these mid-second-trimester fetuses? Figure A (fetus 1) is an axial view of the both kidneys (arrows). Figure B (fetus 2) shows axial (on the reader's left) and coronal views of the left kidney; +'s in the axial view measure the renal pelvis at 11 mm. S = spine.

2. What are the upper limits of normal for the fetal renal pelvis on prenatal ultrasound?

3. What chromosomal anomaly may present with pyelectasis as one of the findings?

4. Name five potential etiologies for fetal renal pyelectasis.

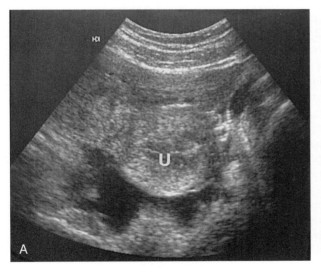

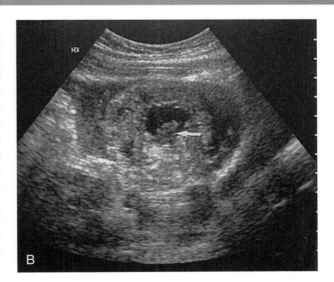

1. In a woman with a positive result on a pregnancy test, what is the diagnosis for these transaxial images of the uterus (Fig. A, U = uterus) and the right adnexa (Fig. B)? What is the arrow pointing to in Figure B?

2. How early does trophoblastic tissue produce β-human chorionic gonadotropin (HCG)?

3. Is the decidual reaction usually normal in the setting of an ectopic pregnancy?

4. What are the sonographic findings following methotrexate therapy to treat an ectopic pregnancy?

C A S E 5 2

Hydronephrosis

1. Fetus 2 (see Fig. B) is abnormal, showing pelvocaliectasis. Fetus 1 (see Fig. A) shows normal mild pyelectasis, without caliectasis.

2. 4 mm or less before 23 weeks' gestation; 7 mm after 23 weeks.

3. Down syndrome (trisomy 21).

4. Vesicoureteral reflux, ureterocele with ureterovesical junction obstruction, ureteropelvic junction obstruction, urethral atresia, and posterior urethral valves.

References

Anderson N, Traci C-E, Allan R, et al: Detection of obstructive uropathy in the fetus: Predictive value of sonographic measurements of renal pelvic diameter at various gestational ages. *AJR Am J Roentgenol* 164:719-723, 1995.

Kaefer M, Peters CA, Retik AB, Benacerraf BB: Increased renal echogenicity: A sonographic sign for differentiating between obstructive and nonobstructive etiologies of in utero bladder distension. *J Urology* 158:1026-1029, 1997.

Cross-Reference

Ultrasound: THE REQUISITES, pp 273-275; 279-286.

Comment

A number of studies have proposed upper limits of normal for fetal renal pelves throughout the gestation. Prior to 23 weeks, the normal renal pelvis can measure up to 4 mm (3 to 5 mm in range). After 23 weeks, many use 7 mm as a cutoff, but the upper limit of normal in some series is up to 10 mm.

The differential diagnosis of dilated renal pelves includes vesicoureteral reflux, ureteropelvic junction obstruction, posterior urethral valves, duplicated renal collecting system, megaloureter, and ureterocele. Approximately 25% of all fetuses with Down syndrome have pyelectasis. Once pyelectasis is detected, it becomes important to attempt to determine if the cause is an obstruction. Obstructed collecting systems show a greater increase in diameter than do nonobstructed kidneys through pregnancy. Therefore, the presence of caliectasis and interval increase are important indicators of an obstruction.

Associated findings that support an obstructive etiology include ureteral dilatation, bladder wall thickening, and oligohydramnios. Increased echogenicity of the kidneys is a confirmatory finding that reflects a long-term obstruction leading to irreversible damage—secondary renal dysplasia.

Notes

C A S E 5 3

Ruptured Ectopic Pregnancy

1. Ruptured ectopic pregnancy. Arrow = an extrauterine embryonic pole.

2. Eight days after conception.

3. No; it is often thinner than normal.

4. An adnexal mass may persist for more than 3 months, even when the β-HCG level is zero.

References

Fleischer AC, Pennell RG, McKee MS, et al: Ectopic pregnancy: Features at transvaginal sonography. *Radiology* 174:375-378, 1990.

Frates MC, Laing FC: Sonographic evaluation of ectopic pregnancy: An update. *AJR Am J Roentgenol* 165:251-259, 1995.

Nyberg DA, Hughes MP, Mack LA, Wang KY: Extrauterine findings of ectopic pregnancy at transvaginal US: Importance of echogenic fluid. *Radiology* 178:823-826, 1991.

Cross-Reference

Ultrasound: THE REQUISITES, pp 415-431.

Comment

This case demonstrates an ectopic gestation diagnosed by transabdominal ultrasound. In most cases, transvaginal ultrasound is required to confirm.

Transvaginal sonography enables detection of several findings that correlate with the presence of an ectopic pregnancy. Sonographic abnormalities can be seen with a β-HCG as low as 30 to 60 mIU/ml. Seventy percent of all unruptured ectopics will have a "tubal ring," a 1- to 3-cm mass with a central hypoechoic area surrounded by concentric hyperechoic tissue (see Fig. B). A tubal ring may be detected even if the tube is ruptured. Intraperitoneal fluid is seen in 63%; echogenic fluid suggests a hemoperitoneum (see Fig. A, posterior to the uterus). Twenty percent of patients with a ruptured tube, however, have no fluid or only a trace of detectable fluid. An extrauterine gestational sac can also be seen.

Methotrexate is being administered with increasing frequency for the treatment of ectopic pregnancy. At our institution, a tubal ring greater than or equal to 2.5 cm is a contraindication to methotrexate and requires laparoscopy or laparotomy for treatment; similarly, signs of a ruptured ectopic or clinical instability would require surgery. Following methotrexate administration, an adnexal mass may transiently enlarge with increased Doppler flow. It is not unusual for the mass to persist for more than 3 months, even after the β-HCG level has declined to zero.

Notes

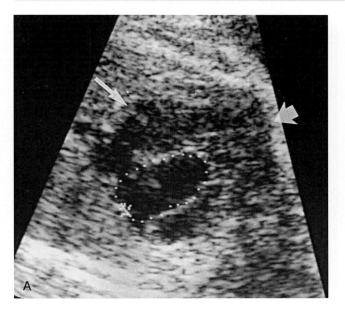

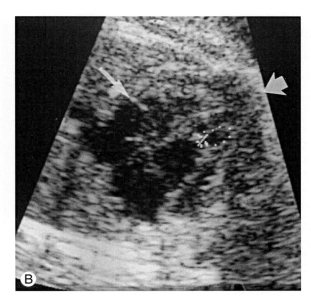

1. On the four-chamber views of a late second-trimester fetal heart, dots outline the fetal right atrium (Fig. A) and right ventricle (Fig. B)? The long arrow denotes the position of the mitral valve. The short arrow marks the cardiac apex. What is the diagnosis?

2. Does the tricuspid valve regurgitate in this anomaly?

3. What is the maternal drug that results in this fetal anomaly?

4. What is the significance of the size of the fossa ovalis in Ebstein's anomaly?

Ebstein's Anomaly

1. Ebstein's anomaly.

2. Yes.

3. Lithium.

4. A small fossa ovalis has a worse prognosis.

References

Pavlova M, Fouron J-C, Susan P, et al: Factors affecting the prognosis of Ebstein's anomaly during fetal life. *Am Heart J* 135:1081–1085, 1998.

Weil SR, Huhta JC: Sonographic differential diagnosis of fetal cardiac abnormalities. *Semin Ultrasound CT MR* 14:298–317, 1993.

Cross-Reference

Ultrasound: THE REQUISITES, pp 238–243.

Comment

Ebstein's anomaly results from displacement of a dysplastic tricuspid valve into the right ventricle, with consequent massive enlargement of the right atrium and atrialized right ventricle. Maternal lithium ingestion during pregnancy is a risk factor. The mortality rate has been quoted to be as high as 85% in the perinatal period, which is considerably worse if the neonate presents with cyanosis.

Fetal ultrasound demonstrates a severely enlarged heart. The right atrium/atrialized right ventricle are greatly dilated (see Fig. A). The true residual right ventricle (see Fig. B) is small. The tricuspid valve is regurgitant, and tricuspid and pulmonic stenosis may also be present. The ductus arteriosus should be interrogated because ductal flow from the aorta to the pulmonary artery predicts postnatal ductal dependence for adequate pulmonary flow, owing to right-to-left shunting of desaturated blood.

Follow-up examinations are performed to measure the size of the chambers throughout the gestation and evaluate for decompensation revealed by hydrops. The true size of the right ventricular cavity is one factor that dictates the ability of the heart to compensate for increased pulmonary blood flow postnatally. Interestingly, left ventricular output affects whether a fetus will reach term without problems. Because the fetal cardiac chambers run in parallel (rather than in a series as the postnatal heart functions) and owing to communications between the great vessels and cardiac atria, the left ventricle may be able to compensate for right ventricular dysfunction.

Notes

Fair Game

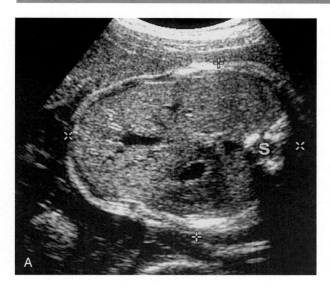

A

1. In a third-trimester ultrasound examination, is this a normal transaxial appearance of the midabdomen (Fig. A)? The side-to-side and anteroposterior dimensions are marked by +'s and x's, respectively. S = spine.

2. Is this an omphalocele? State your reasons.

3. Can ultrasound scanning in the second or third trimester create this appearance?

4. If ultrasound scanning can produce this appearance, can it be corrected?

C A S E 5 5

Pseudo-Omphalocele

1. No.

2. No. The anterior abdominal wall is intact.

3. Yes, if there is undue transducer pressure on the maternal abdomen, transmitted to the fetus, during scanning.

4. Yes, by decreasing the transducer pressure on the maternal abdomen (see Fig. B).

References

Hashimoto BE, Filly RA, Callen PW: Fetal pseudo-ascites: Further anatomic observations. *J Ultrasound Med* 5:151–152, 1986.

Lindfors KK, McGahan JP, Walter JP: Fetal omphalocele and gastroschisis: Pitfalls and sonographic diagnosis. *AJR Am J Roentgenol* 147:797–800, 1986.

Cross-Reference

Ultrasound: THE REQUISITES, p 265.

Comments

The Ultrasound Obstetrical Standards proposed by both the American College of Radiology and the American Institute of Ultrasound in Medicine state that identification of the anterior abdominal wall and cord insertion are part of a routine fetal anatomic survey. When midline defects occur in the anterior abdominal wall, allowing bowel or organs to protrude into an abnormal position, an omphalocele is present. Depending on the size of the defect, this is either at or adjacent to the cord insertion. The protrusions are covered only by a thin amnioperitoneal membrane. Gastroschises constitute an off-midline defect, which occurs commonly in the right lower quadrant. The defect is typically so small that it is often not appreciated; the loops of bowel protruding outside of the fetus can be clearly identified. Rarely, an umbilical hernia may give a small focal bulge at the base of the umbilical cord.

The normal fetal anterior abdominal wall should have a smooth contour with a uniform thickness. The outer layer is a uniformly thick hyperechoic rim (at least 2 mm). Commonly, a hypoechoic layer is identified immediately inside the outer layer and is thought to represent normal intra-abdominal fat (Fig. B; arrows show the hyperechoic outer layer, and the curved arrow indicates the hypoechoic inner layer of the anterior abdominal wall). When these layers are present, regardless of the contour of the anterior abdominal wall, the abdominal wall is normally intact. Nevertheless, the normal anterior abdominal wall is typically round (see Fig. B), and detection of a "pot belly" appearance of the abdomen cannot be considered normal, except if it can be shown that transducer pressure had pincered the fetal body between maternal structures. When this occurs (see Fig. A), the fetal body has a transient bulge that gives the appearance of an omphalocele. Upon releasing the pressure (see Fig. B performed seconds after Fig. A), the body returns to its normal shape. This is a potentially important drawback and is called a pseudo-omphalocele. If not appreciated, an omphalocele could be incorrectly diagnosed. The transducer pressure has not been shown to cause any permanent problems for the fetus.

Note that there is no amniotic fluid between the uterine wall and the fetal abdomen in Figure A during compression, but normal amniotic fluid is present around the body in Figure B once the pressure is released.

Notes

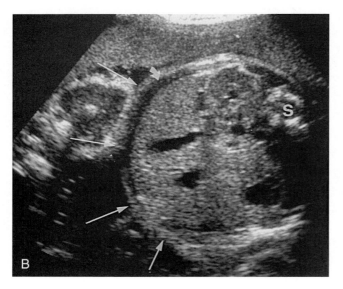

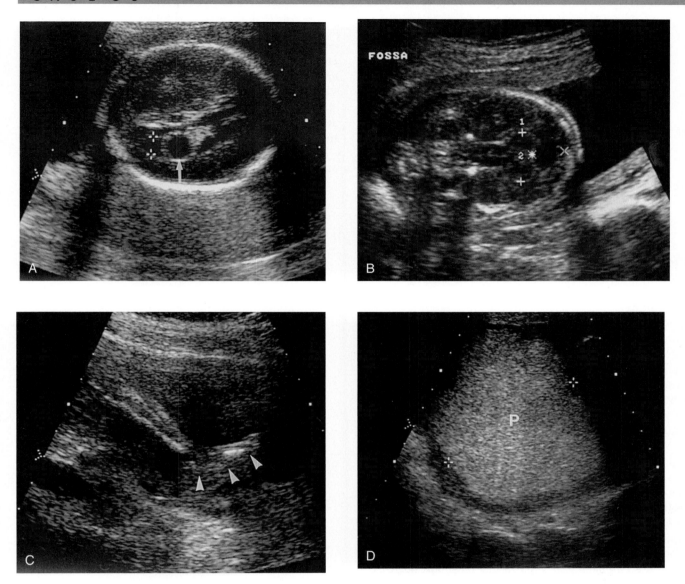

1. In this 28-week-old fetus, what are the two fetal head abnormalities detected by the arrow in Figure A and the x's in Figure B? What is the likely chromosomal anomaly? Figure A is an axial image with +'s measuring the ventricular atrium. Figure B is a slanted axial image used to evaluate the posterior fossa (+'s = the cerebellum).

2. What percentage of cases of this entity have choroid plexus cysts?

3. What limb anomaly is suggested by arrowheads in Figure C of the fetal leg and foot?

4. Which abnormality is denoted by the measurement (+'s) of the placenta (P) in Figure D?

Trisomy 18

1. Figure A; the arrow points to a choroid plexus cyst. Figure B; x's denote an enlarged cisterna magna. Trisomy 18.

2. Choroid plexus cysts are present in 25% to 30% of cases of trisomy 18.

3. Rocker-bottom foot deformity.

4. Enlarged placenta.

Reference

Nyberg DA, Kramer D, Resta R, et al: Prenatal sonographic findings of trisomy 18: Review of 47 cases. *J Ultrasound Med* 2:103–113, 1993.

Cross-Reference

Ultrasound: THE REQUISITES, pp 223; 302–305.

Comment

Trisomy 18 (Edwards' syndrome), comes second to trisomy 21 (Down syndrome) in terms of frequency of autosomal trisomies. Neonates with this disorder do not usually live longer than 1 week. In one series, the meadian survival rate was 3 days. Affected mothers have a bimodal age distribution of 25 to 29 years and 35 to 39 years of age; the prevalence increases with advanced maternal age.

More than 130 associated malformations have been described. Ultrasound can detect abnormalities in 80% of cases, and even a higher percentage of cases if imaging is performed after 24 weeks. Intrauterine growth restriction is seen in almost 90% of cases after 24 weeks. In the setting of polyhydramnios, symmetric intrauterine growth restriction should raise concern regarding trisomy 18.

Cardiac anomalies are present in almost 90% of cases. The most common malformations are atrial septal defect, ventriculoseptal defect, persistent ductus arteriosus, and dysplastic valves. Noncardiac malformations include cystic hygroma and bowel containing omphalocele.

Central nervous system malformations include a "strawberry-shaped" calvarium, which is believed to result from a hypoplastic frontal lobe of the brain. Choroid plexus cysts are present in 25% to 30% of cases (see Fig. A). Between 80% and 90% of fetuses with trisomy 18 and choroid plexus cysts will have at least one other malformation facilitating diagnosis by prenatal ultrasound. Other central nervous system findings include meningomyelocele and an enlarged cisterna magna (see Fig. B). The cisterna magna measured from the posterior margin of the vermis to the inside margin of the occiput (x's) should not measure greater than 10 mm. If present, cisterna magna enlargement is frequently not detected until after 24 weeks. An enlarged cisterna magna without other abnormalities is often normal.

Both upper and lower limb anomalies may be present. Clenched fists, rocker-bottom feet (see Fig. C), and clubbed feet are associated. Decreased fetal movement and overlapping of fingers are attributed to generalized muscle spasticity.

The placenta can be enlarged. A measurement taken at its midpoint, perpendicular to its insertion, should normally be less than 4 cm (see Fig. D, +'s).

Notes

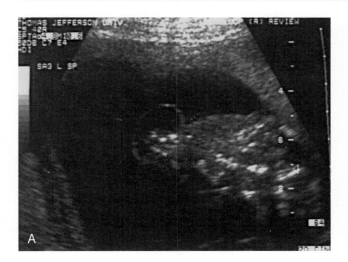

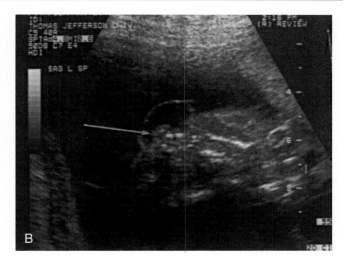

1. What is the differential diagnosis of the abnormality shown in the oblique image of the lower fetal spine (Fig. A)?

2. What spinal finding would aid in the distinction?

3. What abdominal finding would aid in the distinction?

4. Does an elevated α-fetoprotein (AFP) level aid in the distinction?

Myelomeningocele Versus Sacrococcygeal Teratoma

1. Myelomeningocele versus sacrococcygeal teratoma.

2. Splaying or distortion of the posterior elements is compatible with a myelomeningocele.

3. Hydronephrosis may be seen with a sacrococcygeal teratoma (SCT).

4. No.

Reference

Sheth S, Nussbaum SR, Sanders RC, et al: Prenatal diagnosis of sacrococcygeal teratoma: Sonographic-pathologic correlation. *Radiology* 169:131–136, 1988.

Cross-Reference

Ultrasound: THE REQUISITES, pp 228–233.

Comment

This case demonstrates an anechoic mass (myelomeningocele) originating from the dorsum of the lower lumbosacral spine. Although this is typical for a myelomeningocele, a subtype of an SCT may present as a unilocular cystic mass.

Associated findings with a myelomeningocele include splayed or distorted posterior elements of the spine (Fig. B, arrow), hydrocephalus, banana-shaped cerebellum, and lemon-head deformity of the calvarium (Chiari malformation). SCT may result in displacement of the bladder and hydronephrosis owing to an anterior (presacral) component. Hydronephrosis is a poor prognostic indicator. An elevated AFP level may be present in both cases, because immature components (yolk sac tumor components) of an SCT may secrete AFP.

Notes

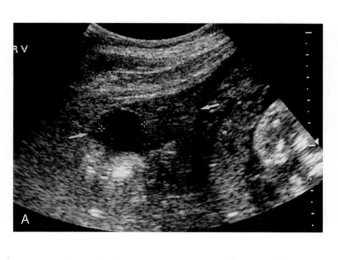

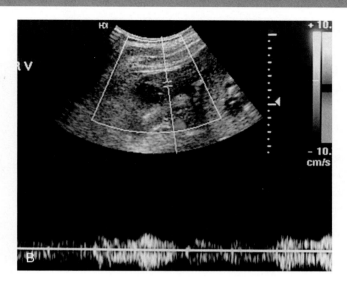

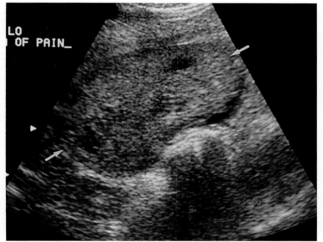

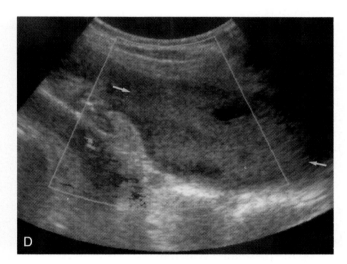

1. What is the abnormality in this 20-year-old pregnant patient with cyclical left-sided pelvic pain? Figures A and B display the right ovary. Figure B indicates a spectral Doppler signal from the soft tissue of that ovary (arrows = the ovary; +'s = a simple follicle). Figures C and D illustrate the left ovary (arrows = the ovary). Figure D provides a color Doppler evaluation.

2. What is the typical age (stage of life) of a patient with this diagnosis?

3. List three risk factors.

4. Is Doppler analysis a reliable aid in the diagnosis of this entity?

C A S E 5 8

Ovarian Torsion

1. Left ovarian torsion.

2. Premenopausal.

3. Ovarian mass, ovarian hyperstimulation syndrome, and pregnancy.

4. No.

References
Lee EJ, Kwon HC, Joo HJ, et al: Diagnosis of ovarian torsion with color Doppler sonography: Depiction of the twisted vascular pedicle. *J Ultrasound Med* 17:83–89, 1998.

Stark JE, Siegel MJ: Ovarian torsion in prepubertal and pubertal girls: Sonographic findings. *AJR Am J Roentgenol* 163:1479–1482, 1994.

Cross-Reference
Ultrasound: THE REQUISITES, pp 407, 413.

Comment
Ovarian torsion is a cause of acute abdominal pain in women that requires rapid diagnosis and treatment. Torsion occurs most commonly in women of reproductive years; a nonadherent ipsilateral adnexal mass is present in 50% to 81% of cases, most commonly a benign teratoma. Nonetheless, torsion of the normal ovary can occur in prepubertal females because of adnexal mobility. Ovarian torsion is slightly more common on the right side. Risk factors include the presence of an adnexal mass, ovarian hyperstimulation syndrome, and pregnancy. The pain is classically cyclical and grows worse with each cycle, although constant or vague pain may be the presenting symptom.

The appearance of ovarian torsion has been described with ultrasound, computed tomography, and magnetic resonance imaging. With ultrasound, the findings vary depending on the age of the patient. However, an enlarged ovary or mass should be present as the lead point of the torsion (see Fig. C). The appearance of a torsed ovary is variable, depending on whether an underlying mass is present and the degree of hemorrhage or necrosis, resulting in cystic and hyperechoic components. Free fluid is present in up to two thirds of cases.

Color and pulsed Doppler ultrasound have been shown to be unreliable in the definitive diagnosis of ovarian torsion. Whereas an enlarged abnormal appearing ovary with no arterial or venous flow may indicate torsion (see Fig. D), arterial and venous flow have been demonstrated in surgically proven cases of ovarian torsion. Therefore, the persistence of blood flow depends on the degree of torsion. Arterial flow with no diastolic component or absence of venous flow can be seen early. Venous thrombosis may precede arterial occlusion.

The twisted vascular pedicle is defined as the rotation site of the ovarian pedicle and has been imaged with ultrasound. The pedicle was located either adjacent to the ovary/ovarian mass or between the ovary and the uterus, where vessels usually run in a straight course. In cases where flow was still identified in the twisted pedicle, the ovary was viable at surgery and the pedicle was untwisted. The patients with no flow had necrotic ovaries.

Notes

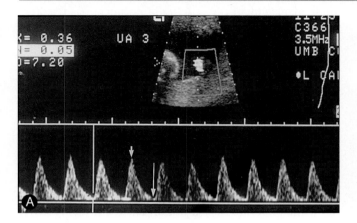
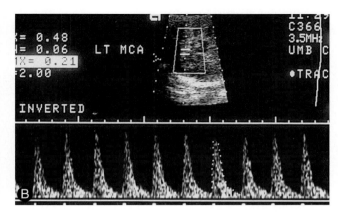

1. What does decreased, absent, or reversed diastolic flow in the umbilical artery indicate (Fig. A)?

2. What is the purpose of measuring the flow of the middle cerebral artery (MCA) (Fig. B)?

3. How is the umbilical artery impedance measured?

4. What is the normal pattern of the umbilical artery Doppler as the gestation progresses?

Umbilical Artery Doppler

1. Placental insufficiency and possibly a fetal abnormality.

2. To determine whether a compensatory, brain-sparing fetal response has occurred in response to decreased umbilical artery diastolic flow.

3. As a ratio of peak systolic velocity (short arrow) divided by end-diastolic velocity (long arrow) (systolic/diastolic [S/D] ratio) (see Fig. A).

4. Increasing diastolic flow (lower ratio).

References

Alfirevic Z, Neilson JP: Fetus-placenta-newborn: Doppler ultrasonography in high-risk pregnancies: Systematic review with meta-analysis. *Am J Obstet Gynecol* 172:1379–1387, 1995.

Sepulveda W, Shennan A, Peek MJ: Reverse end-diastolic flow in the middle cerebral artery: An agonal pattern in the human fetus. *Am J Obstet Gynecol* 174:1645–1647, 1996.

Valcamonico A, Danti L, Frusca T, et al: Absent end-diastolic velocity in umbilical artery: Risk of neonatal morbidity and brain damage. *Am J Obstet Gynecol* 170:796–801, 1994.

Cross-Reference

Ultrasound: THE REQUISITES, pp 185–187.

Comment

Doppler ultrasound has become an important component in the prenatal evaluation of high-risk pregnancies. The umbilical artery waveform can indicate abnormal fetal-placental blood flow by demonstrating elevated placental impedance. An abnormal umbilical artery waveform is associated with a higher incidence of adverse fetal outcome.

Indications for measuring the umbilical artery waveform include the presence of oligohydramnios and intrauterine growth restriction. A waveform should be obtained from the fetal end of the cord and also from the middle and the maternal end of the cord. The S/D ratio (peak systolic velocity/end-diastolic velocity) at each of these three points is averaged and compared with a chart of normal values for each gestational age (see Fig. A). With increasing gestational age, the S/D ratio should decrease, reflecting decreasing impedance.

If the impedance increases, the diastolic flow will decrease and can be absent or reversed (see Fig. A). Absence or reversal of diastolic flow has been associated with intrauterine growth restriction, fetal asphyxia, perinatal mortality, and long-term permanent fetal neurologic sequelae. In addition, there is a higher likelihood that the fetus has a chromosomal anomaly. Routine use of the Doppler ultrasound of the umbilical artery to guide management (i.e., timing of delivery) has resulted in a lower incidence of antenatal admissions, labor induction, emergent cesarean section for fetal distress, perinatal death, and hypoxic fetal encephalopathy.

When fetal hypoxia results from decreased diastolic umbilical artery flow, the fetal circulation responds with a "brain-sparing" effect. The MCA index is measured either as the S/D ratio or as a pulsatility index [that is peak systole minus end-diastole divided by the area of one waveform] (see Fig. B, the dotted lines outline one waveform). The MCA Doppler is evaluated to determine if blood is being redistributed from other sources (i.e., mesenteric) to the intracranial structures. In this case, the MCA pulsatility index is normal, reflecting redistribution of blood to the brain (see Fig. B). If further decompensation occurs, the MCA pulsatility index actually *decreases*, and diastolic flow to the brain increases.

Notes

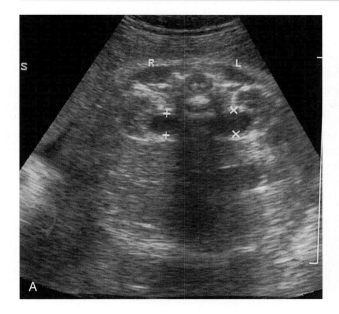

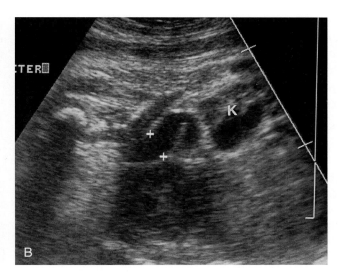

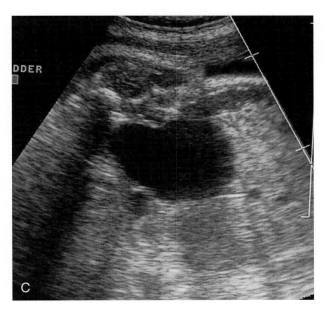

1. What are the findings and the differential diagnoses in this third-trimester fetus? Figure A is an axial view of the fetal kidneys (+'s = renal pelves; R = right kidney; L = left kidney). Figure B is a coronal image of the lower abdomen (K = left kidney; +'s = ureter). Figure C is an oblique image of the fetal pelvis.

2. What two findings aid in confirming that dilatation of the renal collecting system is obstructive?

3. What is the classic appearance of the bladder with posterior urethral valves (PUVs)?

4. Does dilatation of the renal collecting system always indicate an obstruction?

C A S E 6 0

Posterior Urethral Valves

1. Dilated urinary tract from the kidneys to the bladder. The differential diagnoses are posterior urethral valves (male), urethral agenesis (female), prune-belly syndrome, and megacystis-megaureter syndrome.

2. Bladder wall thickening and echogenic (hyperechoic) kidneys.

3. Keyhole.

4. No.

References

Hutton KAR, Thomas DFM, Davies BW: Prenatally detected posterior urethral valves: Qualitative assessment of second trimester scans and prediction of outcome. *J Urol* 158:1022–1025, 1997.

Kaefer M, Peters CA, Retik AB, Benacerraf BB: Increased renal echogenicity: A sonographic sign for differentiating between obstructive and nonobstructive etiologies of in utero bladder distension. *J Urol* 158:1026–1029, 1997.

Cross-Reference
Ultrasound: THE REQUISITES, pp 278–283.

Comment
Detection of an enlarged fetal bladder immediately raises the concern for an obstructive etiology. The fetus should be imaged over time to determine if the bladder will empty; the bladder fills and empties every 15 to 45 minutes. Bladder dilatation can be caused by obstructive etiologies (e.g., posterior urethral valves in males, urethral atresia in females) or nonobstructive etiologies (e.g., prune-belly syndrome, megacystis-megaureter syndrome). Dilatation of the pelvicaliceal system (hydronephrosis) and ureter (hydroureter) can be caused by obstructive etiologies (e.g., posterior urethral valves, urethral atresia, ectopic ureterocele) or by nonobstructive etiologies (e.g., prune-belly syndrome, megacystis-megaureter syndrome, vesicoureteral reflux).

Determining fetal gender is important in cases of urinary tract obstruction. In a male fetus, the most likely diagnosis in this case is an obstructive uropathy secondary to PUVs, which occurs exclusively in males (see Figs. A to C). A keyhole appearance of the urinary bladder is classic for PUVs (Fig. D, arrows).

The timing of detection and the degree of obstruction have been shown to be predictors of outcome in fetuses with PUVs. An obstructed bladder detected before 28 weeks carries a poor prognosis. Obstruction of the urinary tract that results in dilatation detected at this early age often results in intrauterine death or poor renal function in those who survive. With moderate to severe upper tract dilatation, the prognosis is significantly worse than with isolated bladder distention or mild upper tract dilatation. Moderate to severe dilatation is defined as the anteroposterior diameter of the renal pelvis of 10 mm or greater with caliectasis. Detection of echogenic kidneys or cystic renal parenchymal changes indicate renal dysplasia, which also has a poor prognosis.

In utero decompression can be performed with vesicoamniotic shunting. However, this has not been shown to improve outcome. Nonetheless, detection of the posterior urethral valves and characterization of the degree of obstruction may be helpful in counseling parents about the prognosis.

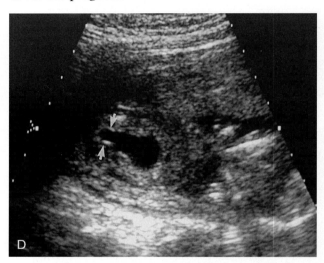

Notes

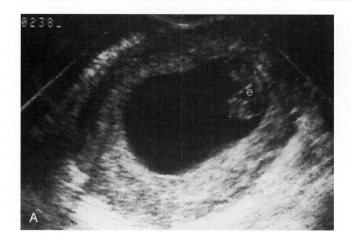

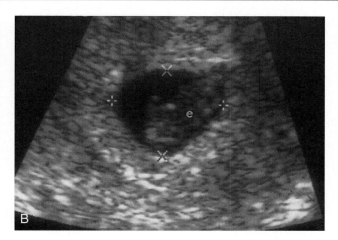

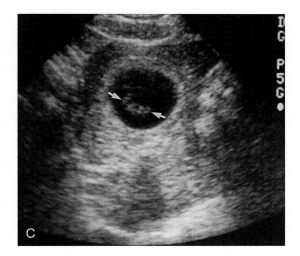

1. Which of these early pregnancies is normal (Figs. A to C; embryos = e or arrows)? Why?

2. At what size of a gestational sac size should you visualize: (1) a yolk sac, and (2) a fetal pole transvaginally?

3. Can the detection of a yolk sac in the first trimester predict pregnancy as an outcome?

4. Does detection of an embryo less than 5 mm in size without a heartbeat indicate fetal demise?

Early Intrauterine Gestational Sac

1. Figure C is normal. The normal gestational sac is about twice the length of the embryo with appropriate surrounding fluid. In the other two, the gestational sac is too large (see Fig. A) and too small (see Fig. B) for the embryo.

2. The yolk sac should be seen with an 8-mm sac; the fetal pole should be seen with a 12-mm sac. If they do not meet these criteria, follow-up is advised as long as the gestational sac appears to be normal. Normal intrauterine pregnancies (IUPs) are occasionally delayed, and an embryo is not detected until the gestational sac is approximately 20 mm.

3. No.

4. No.

References

Bree RL, Edwards M, Bohm-Velez M, et al: Transvaginal sonography in the evaluation of normal early pregnancy: Correlation with HCG Level. *AJR Am J Roentgenol* 153:75–79, 1989.

Kurtz AB, Needleman L, Pennell RG, et al: Can detection of the yolk sac in the first trimester be used to predict the outcome of pregnancy? *AJR Am J Roentgenol* 158:843–847, 1992.

Mehta RS, Levine D, Beckwith B: Treatment of ectopic pregnancy: Is a human chorionic gonadotropin level of 2000 mIU/ml a reasonable threshold? *Radiology* 205:569–573, 1997.

Cross-Reference
Ultrasound: THE REQUISITES, pp 191–203.

Comment

Many ultrasound imaging criteria have been described to aid in distinguishing a normal IUP from an abnormal IUP or anembryonic gestation. It is essential to know the quantitative β-human chorionic gonadotropin (β-HCG) level when evaluating any early pregnancy. Also, you must know which international standard (IS) is being performed in your laboratory. There are three different tests: the first, second, and third IS. The first IS is twice the second IS. The third IS is 1.8 times the second IS (similar to the first).

Data suggested that an intrauterine sac should be visible by 1000 mIU/ml using the first and third IS. Accordingly, in cases where the BHCE level is 1000–2000 mIU/ml and no IUP is seen with transvaginal ultrasound, ectopic pregnancy becomes a concern. However, a recent study has shown that in cases where no definite IUP was visible by transvaginal ultrasound with a β-HCG of 2000 mIU/ml, normal pregnancies subsequently developed in 1/3 of cases. It is essential to be careful when interpreting these studies, because methotrexate is being administered with increasing frequency by obstetricians if an ectopic pregnancy is suspected when no IUP is visible by ultrasound. Close follow-up should be considered if clinically appropriate.

Once an early sac is identified in the uterus, transvaginal scanning is often required to visualize a yolk sac or a small fetal pole. A yolk sac should be visible when the sac is 8 mm; the fetal pole should be visible when the sac is 12 mm. However, follow-up should be recommended as a normal IUP may be identified later even when these criteria are not met; some embryos are not visualized until the gestational sac exceeds 18 mm.

The yolk sac becomes visible before the fetal pole. The presence of a yolk sac is not consistently predictive of a normal early pregnancy. The absence of a yolk sac does not necessarily indicate a miscarriage. If a fetal pole is seen, fetal heart motion is usually detected when the fetal pole is equal to or greater than 5 mm. The size of the fetal pole in relation to the sac is also predictive of the outcome. If the fetal pole is too small for the sac (see Fig. A) or too large for the sac (see Fig. B), fetal demise often results.

Notes

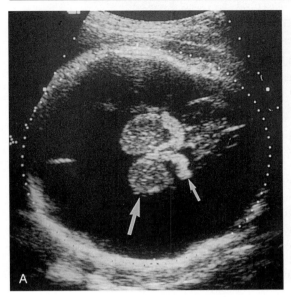

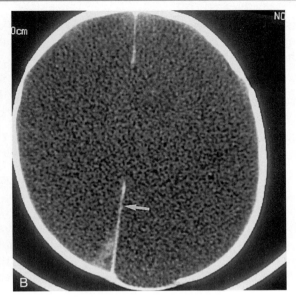

1. From this axial ultrasound image of a third-trimester fetus (Fig. A), what is the most likely diagnosis? Name the labeled structures.
2. Name the structure labeled in the neonatal computed tomography (CT) scan of the head (Fig. B, arrow). What diagnosis does it exclude?
3. Would ventricular shunting be indicated in this case?
4. What is the presumed etiology of this disorder?

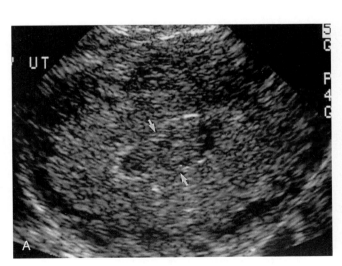

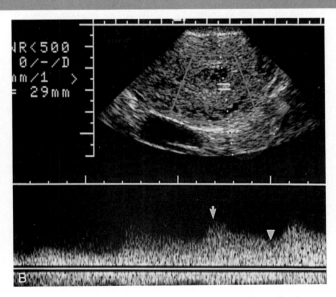

1. This 22-year-old woman presents with vaginal bleeding after a miscarriage (spontaneous abortion) (Figs. A and B). Figure A is a transvaginal axial/coronal image of the uterus (arrows = a 15-mm endometrial thickness). What is your most likely diagnosis?
2. Can a molar pregnancy (hydatidiform mole) present with a similar appearance?
3. What is the normal endometrial thickness following a miscarriage (spontaneous abortion) or a dilatation and curettage?
4. How can Doppler ultrasound help in the evaluation of the uterine findings (see Fig. B)? Figure B displays a split-screen image of the same patient; the upper half shows the uterus with a pulsed Doppler cursor in the endometrium, and the lower half shows the spectral waveform (arrow = peak systole; arrowhead = end-diastole).

Hydranencephaly

1. Hydranencephaly. Large arrow = thalamus; small arrow = choroid plexus.

2. Falx; alobar holoprosencephaly.

3. No; shunting is indicated for noncommunicating or obstructive hydrocephalus.

4. Bilateral internal carotid artery (ICA) infarctions. Infection has also been associated.

Reference

Greene MF, Benaceraff BR, Crawford JM: Hydranencephaly: US appearance during in utero evolution. *Radiology* 156:779–780, 1985.

Cross-Reference

Ultrasound: THE REQUISITES, pp 213–214.

Comment

Hydranencephaly is caused by massive bilateral cortical destruction with ex vacuo enlargement of the already formed lateral ventricles. Leptomeninges surround fluid replacing the cerebral cortex. Remaining structures include the brainstem, thalami, cerebellum, and choroid plexus, which continues to make cerebrospinal fluid, accounting for the associated macrocephaly.

The etiology is believed by many to be the result of a bilateral supraclinoid ICA infarct. In addition to the proposed etiology of an ICA infarct, infection is believed to be the cause in some cases. Associated infections include toxoplasmosis, herpes virus, equine virus, and cytomegalic virus inclusion disease.

A prenatal ultrasound distinction from marked hydrocephalus is essential but often difficult to make. Identification of a thin mantle of residual cerebral cortex confirms that hydrocephalus is the etiology. The presence of the falx (arrow in Fig. B) and separate thalami (large arrow in Fig. A) distinguish hydranencephaly from alobar holoprosencephaly. The face is normal in hydranencephaly, as opposed to the various facial anomalies associated with holoprosencephaly. Polyhydramnios is usually present in conjunction with hydranencephaly as well as the other central nervous system malformations.

The disorder usually leads to death in the first few days of life; rarely, a child will live several months or longer. Postnatal CT is helpful in evaluating suspected hydranencephaly. Massive subdural effusions may mimic hydranencephaly on postnatal CT.

Notes

Retained Products of Conception

1. Retained products of conception (POCs).

2. Unlikely, because the amount of tissue is small; furthermore, the tissue does not have good through-transmission.

3. No greater than 5 mm.

4. Doppler ultrasound helps to distinguish retained POCs from decidua and hemorrhage.

References

Hertzberg BS, Bowie JD: Ultrasound of the postpartum uterus: Prediction of retained placental tissue. *J Ultrasound Med* 10:451–456, 1991.

Kurtz AB, Shlaansky-Goldberg RD, Choi HY, et al: Detection of retained products of conception following spontaneous abortion in the first trimester. *J Ultrasound Med* 10:387–395, 1991.

Cross-Reference

Ultrasound: THE REQUISITES, pp 367–371.

Comment

On ultrasound, retained POCs may be difficult to distinguish from intrauterine decidua, hemorrhage, and endometrium. Following a spontaneous abortion or after a dilatation and curettage, an endometrial stripe of less than 5 mm in thickness is an excellent but not absolute predictor of the *absence* of a retained POC. Any endometrial collection or endometrial thickening greater than 5 mm suggests retained POCs. The endometrial contents may appear as hypoechoic or hyperechoic solid material, with or without a mass; heterogeneous fluid with solid material; or a solid mass with calcification. A hyperechoic mass (>15 mm) that expands the endometrial canal is the best predictor (see Fig. A, arrows).

The differential diagnosis should also include a molar pregnancy (hydatidiform mole), which may also present with vaginal bleeding. On ultrasound examination, this tissue may be hyperechoic, as in this case; however, owing to the multiple fluid-filled spaces, the tissue will have good through-transmission. The uterus is usually very enlarged.

Active trophoblastic tissue from any source will give arterial waveforms with elevated diastolic flow (low impedance) (see Fig. B). When detected, it distinguishes retained POCs from decidua and hemorrhage. However, similar waveforms can be seen with a hydatidiform mole. The serum β-human chorionic gonadotropin levels will be persistently elevated with a molar pregnancy, but low or even falling with POCs.

Notes

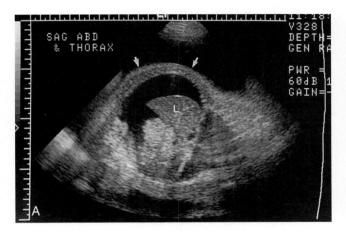

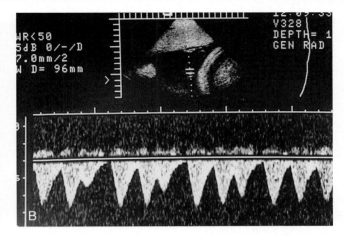

1. What are the findings in this third-trimester fetus and what is the diagnosis (Fig. A)? Figure A is a sagittal image of the fetal body. The thorax lies toward the reader's right. L = liver; arrows = the anterior abdominal wall.

2. Can Doppler ultrasound of the umbilical artery establish a cause for the appearance of this fetus (Fig. B)?

3. What is believed to be one of the earliest findings if this presents in the first trimester?

4. What is the outcome?

Nonimmune Fetal Hydrops

1. Ascites and skin thickening. Fetal hydrops (hydrops fetalis).

2. Yes; nonimmune hydrops, caused by fetal tachyarrhythmia (trigeminy).

3. Increased nuchal translucency.

4. Poor; mortality is higher than 70%.

References

Jauniaux E: Diagnosis and management of early nonimmune hydrops fetalis. *Prenat Diagn* 17:1261–1268, 1997.

Santolaya J, Jaffe R, Warsof SL: Antenatal classification of hydrops fetalis. *Obstet Gynecol* 79:256–259, 1992.

Cross-Reference

Ultrasound: THE REQUISITES, pp 243–245.

Comment

Fetal hydrops (hydrops fetalis) is a condition of fluid accumulation in the fetal pleural, peritoneal, and pericardial spaces as well as skin edema and placentomegaly (see Fig. A). At present, isoimmunization related to blood group incompatibilities of the mother and fetus has become a relatively rare cause, and most cases are classified as nonimmune hydrops.

There are approximately 80 different causes of nonimmune hydrops. In the first trimester, this is usually due to a chromosomal defect (e.g., trisomy 21, 18, and 13 or Turner's syndrome) in which lymphatic obstruction causes hydrops. Some believe that increased nuchal translucency is the first manifestation of fluid accumulation due to hydrops. This can be detected as early as 9 weeks, with a nuchal translucency of more than 3 mm. In cases diagnosed during the first trimester, karyotypically normal fetuses have demonstrated resolution of the hydrops later in the gestation. However, the outcome of these fetuses remains unfavorable. If diagnosed before 20 weeks, the two most common indicators of hydrops include generalized skin thickening and placental enlargement.

Structural anomalies account for many cases of hydrops diagnosed after 15 weeks. Common causes include cardiac malformations and cardiac arrhythmias (see Fig. B, tachyarrhythmia), which can be intermittent and not appreciated on any one examination. Other nonimmune cases include cystic hygroma with diffuse lymphatic obstruction and any mass that obstructs venous return to the heart. Teratomas, particularly sacrococcygeal, may lead to hydrops, which is believed to be caused by high outflow through the tumor. The high-output heart failure associated with a vein of Galen arteriovenous malformation or severe anemia are additional causes. Finally, maternal-fetal infection, such as the TORCH (*t*oxoplasmosis, *o*ther infections, *r*ubella, *c*ytomegalovirus, *h*erpes) group and parvovirus can result in hydrops. There is a long list of causes of hydrops, for which we refer you to Nyberg's *Diagnostic Ultrasound of Fetal Anomalies*.

The early detection of fetal hydrops is often difficult. This, however, is important clinically because by the time that fluid is detected within body cavities and marked skin thickening is noted, the fetus is often significantly compromised. Work on fetuses at risk for immune hydrops have found that the length of the liver (from the dome of the right hemidiaphragm to the distal tip) increased as the first sign of impending hydrops in moderate to severe cases. It has not been determined whether this is a uniform finding, and its use in nonimmune hydrops has not been fully worked out.

At present, the outcome of fetus with full-blown sonographic signs of fetal hydrops is generally poor, and mortality is higher than 70%.

Notes

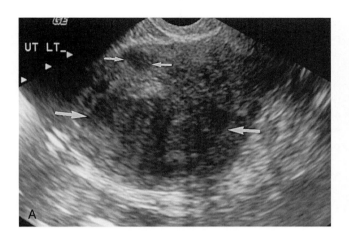

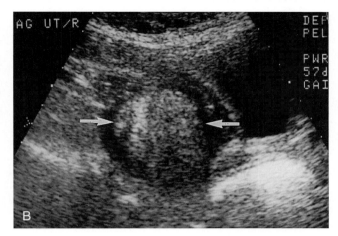

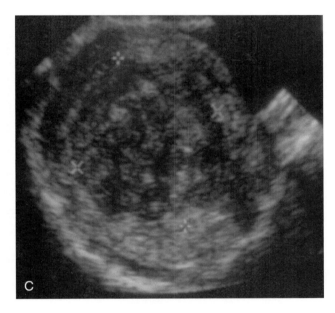

1. Three women present with uterine enlargement and palpable uterine masses (Figs. A to C, denoted by arrows in Figs. A and B and by +'s and x's in Fig. C). One case is a fibroid, one a lipoleiomyoma, and one a leiomyosarcoma. Can you tell them apart?

2. What accounts for the increased echogenicity in the lipoleiomyoma (see Fig. B)?

3. What is the incidence of uterine sarcomas?

4. How is a leiomyosarcoma of the uterus distinguished from a leiomyoma?

Uterine Masses

1. Figure A has two hypoechoic solid masses (arrows) that were fibroids. Figure B, which shows a marked hyperechoic solid mass, was a lipoleiomyoma. Figure C, which is a large heterogeneous solid mass, could have been a fibroid but was a leiomyosarcoma at pathology.

2. Multiple closely packed boundary interfaces of multiple tissue types.

3. 1% to 3% of all uterine malignancies.

4. Often it cannot be distinguished.

References

Cacciatore B, Lehtovirta P, Wahlstrom T, Ylostalo P: Ultrasound findings in uterine mixed müllerian sarcomas and endometrial stromal sarcomas. *Gynecol Oncol* 35:290–293, 1989.

Carter JR, Ruhr DM, Okagaki T, Fowler JM: Uterine lipoleiomyoma: A rare tumor. *J Ultrasound Med* 12:491–492, 1993.

Cross-Reference

Ultrasound: THE REQUISITES, pp 374–378.

Comment

The three uterine masses depicted in this case have different histologic features. Case A shows typical uterine leiomyomas (see Fig. A). These benign masses of smooth muscle are actually monoclonal proliferations of muscle cells. They can be found in subserosal, myometrial, submucosal, or intracavitary locations. On ultrasound, a simple leiomyoma is hypoechoic and solid with some attenuation of the sound beam. The echogenicity may be heterogeneous owing to the presence of calcification, necrosis, hemorrhage, or hyalinization. It is important to describe the relationship with the endometrial lining, and follow-up studies are often performed to evaluate for a change in size.

The mass in Case B is a rare lipoleiomyoma (see Fig. B). This benign subtype of leiomyoma contains lipid. The presence of multiple closely packed boundary interfaces in the tumor (multiple boundary interfaces) account for the homogeneous increased echogenicity on ultrasound. It is important when imaging an exophytic lipoleiomyoma to be certain that the mass arises from the myometrium, because the appearance is similar to that of an ovarian dermoid.

The third case is a uterine leiomyosarcoma (see Fig. C). This rare uterine malignancy can be indistinguishable from a leiomyoma by ultrasound and computed tomography imaging. A rapid increase in size of a leiomyoma should raise concern regarding a leiomyosarcoma. In addition, these masses are usually necrotic and large. The leiomyosarcoma is the most common type of uterine myometrial malignancy. The mixed mesodermal tumor is less common. A characteristic ultrasound appearance of the mixed mesodermal tumor has been described. A heterogeneous myometrial echotexture can be seen with hyperechoic areas and anechoic areas, which may be large and irregularly shaped, scattered throughout the myometrium. Although uterine sarcomas in general have the worst prognosis of uterine masses, the mixed mesodermal tumor has a very poor prognosis.

Notes

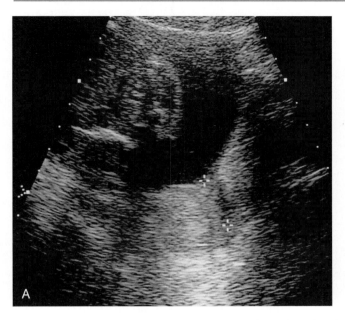
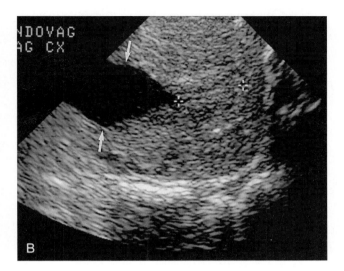

1. Which abnormality is demonstrated in this third-trimester pregnancy by the sagittal images of the lower uterine segment, Figure A (transabdominal) followed by Figure B (transvaginal)? The +'s in both images depict a closed endocervical length of 1.8 cm.

2. What is cervical funneling?

3. Does the shape of the funnel have any significance?

4. Which is more accurate for measuring the cervix—ultrasound or a digital examination?

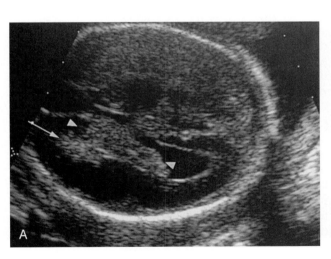
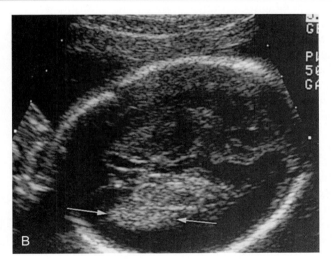

1. Which abnormality is shown in these axial images of a late second-trimester fetal brain (Figs. A and B, arrows and arrowheads)?

2. Is there a difference in prognosis if this occurs intraventricularly or intraparenchymally?

3. What is the most common cause of this abnormality?

4. At what time in the gestation is this usually detected?

Incompetent Cervix

1. Incompetent cervix with funneling.

2. Opening of the internal os. Figure B (arrows).

3. Yes; V-shaped is worse.

4. Ultrasound.

References

Gomez R, Galasso M, Romero R, et al: Ultrasonographic examination of the uterine cervix is better than cervical digital examination as a predictor of the likelihood of premature delivery in patients with preterm labor and intact membranes. *Am J Obstet Gynecol* 171:956–964, 1994.

Iams JD, Goldenberg RL, Meis PJ, et al: The length of the cervix and the risk of spontaneous premature delivery. *N Engl J Med* 334:567–572, 1996.

Cross-Reference

Ultrasound: THE REQUISITES, pp 329–333.

Comment

It is well established that cervical shortening is associated with preterm delivery. Although many observers believe that an endocervical length between 2.5 and 3 cm is the lower limits of normal, there is a continuum. A normal cervical length is 3 cm or more; 2 to 3 cm is borderline; and less than 2 cm is definitely abnormal (see Figs. A and B).

The risk of preterm labor increases gradually as the cervical length shortens. Transvaginal ultrasound has been shown to be a safe and accurate method to measure the cervix. Ultrasound is more accurate than the digital examination, particularly for the detection of opening of the internal os, called funneling. In addition to cervical shortening, a change in cervical length between examinations (particularly a change of 6 mm or more) has a small association with preterm labor.

Funneling is defined as dilatation of the internal os (see Fig. B; arrows = the internal os). The degree of dilatation of the internal os, which defines incompetence, has been quoted as greater than 3 to 6 mm, depending on the source. The length of the funnel has prognostic value. V-shaped funneling has been shown to be more predictive of preterm delivery than has U-shaped funneling.

Transvaginal scanning with an empty bladder is the most consistently accurate technique to evaluate the cervix. The vaginal probe is inserted into the anterior fornix of the vagina, withdrawn slightly, and then advanced only enough to obtain a clear image. This action decreases the pressure on the cervix, which can artificially increase the length.

Notes

Intracranial Hemorrhage

1. Intracranial hemorrhage.

2. Yes.

3. Direct maternal abdominal trauma in the third trimester.

4. Third trimester.

Reference

Vergani P, Strobelt N, Locatelli A, et al: Clinical significance of fetal intracranial hemorrhage. *Am J Obstet Gynecol* 175:536–543, 1996.

Cross-Reference

Ultrasound: THE REQUISITES, pp 224–225.

Comment

Fetal hemorrhage is included in the differential diagnosis of an intracranial fetal mass. In the neonate, changes in cerebral blood pressure and perinatal asphyxia contribute to the development of cerebral hemorrhage. However, in the fetus, the intracerebral pressure is regulated and protected from fluctuations in the maternal blood pressure, which suggests that an alternative pathophysiology might be associated with a cerebral hemorrhage. The most common cause is secondary to direct maternal abdominal trauma in the third trimester. Most hemorrhages are detected after 23 weeks and are possibly related to the fact that the germinal matrix vascular connections to subependymal venous networks develop after 20 weeks.

Prenatal cerebral hemorrhage can occur in the ventricle (arrowheads in Fig. A), parenchyma (arrows in Figs. A and B), or subdural or subarachnoid space. The prognosis is poor with subdural and parenchymal hemorrhages but better in cases of isolated intraventricular hemorrhage. Higher degrees of ventricular dilatation (>15 mm) also worsen the prognosis.

On ultrasound, hemorrhage appears as a hyperechoic (either homogeneous or heterogeneous) mass. Intraventricular hemorrhage may present as an irregular, enlarged choroid plexus. The ventricular diameter and any parenchymal abnormality must be evaluated and closely followed. Magnetic resonance imaging may be helpful in the characterization and delineation of the hemorrhage.

Notes

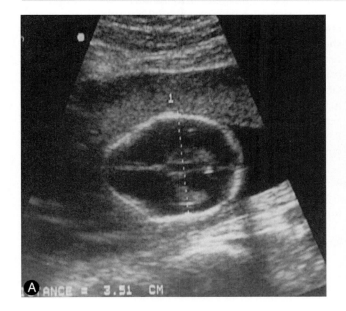

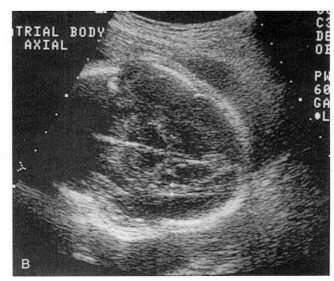

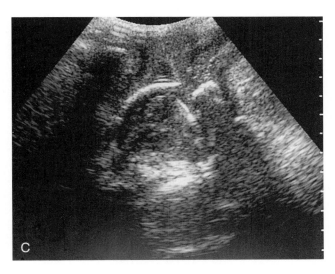

1. Which entity is associated with a "strawberry-shaped skull"?

2. What are the most common central nervous system (CNS) malformations associated with a "lemon head" (Fig. A)?

3. Which syndrome can be associated with a "cloverleaf skull" (Fig. B)?

4. What is Spalding's sign (Fig. C)?

Calvarial Abnormalities

1. Trisomy 18.

2. Myelomeningocele with associated Chiari II malformation; encephalocele.

3. Thanatophoric dwarf.

4. Overlapping fetal skull bones occurring in a second- or third-trimester fetal demise.

References

Ball RH, Filly RA, Goldstein RB, Callen PW: The lemon sign: Not a specific indicator of meningomyelocele. *J Ultrasound Med* 3:131–134, 1993.

Nicolaides KH, Salvesen DR, Snijders RJ, Gosden CM: Strawberry-shaped skull in fetal trisomy 18. *Fetal Diagn Ther* 7:132–137, 1992.

Shiroyama Y, Ito H, Yamashita T, et al: The relationship of cloverleaf skull to hydrocephalus. *Childs Nervous System* 7:382–385, 1991.

Cross-Reference

Ultrasound: THE REQUISITES, pp 230–232; 302.

Comment

Evaluation of the fetal skull begins with a measurement of the biparietal diameter (BPD). This is used to calculate the mean estimated gestational age if the first study is performed at 12 weeks of gestation or later. For follow-up examinations, the gestational age is always dictated by the first study, and the BPD, abdominal circumference and femur length are measured to assess for interval growth. Beyond measuring the BPD, the shape of the fetal skull should be evaluated. Several syndromes have been associated with skull abnormalities.

The "lemon head" (Fig. A) (seen before 24 weeks' gestational age) is a well-known finding in Chiari II malformation: myelomeningocele with a small posterior fossa and a banana-shaped cerebellum. However, one series demonstrated that a lemon-shaped head can be seen in fetuses with other CNS malformations, including encephalocele, Dandy-Walker malformation, and agenesis of the corpus callosum. In addition, a few cases with unrelated anomalies presented with a lemon-shaped head (umbilical vein varix with a two-vessel cord and fetal hydronephrosis); if the deformity is mild, it may be a normal variant.

A "strawberry-shaped" calvarium can be seen in trisomy 18. Although not present in all cases, it is considered to be secondary to hypoplasia of the frontal lobes of the brain. Choroid plexus cysts may also be present. Limb anomalies include rocker-bottom feet, clubbed feet, and overlapping fingers.

A cloverleaf skull or "kleeblattschädel" can be seen in some cases of thanatophoric dwarfism, where it is associated with a narrow, bell-shaped thorax and shortened "telephone receiver"–shaped femurs. However, as shown in Figure B, it can also be due to an isolated craniosynostosis. Additionally, several rare syndromes may involve a cloverleaf skull deformity, including infants with atypical Apert's syndrome, the syndrome of marfanoid phenotype with craniosynostosis (Shprintzen-Goldberg syndrome), and Pfeiffer's syndrome type 2. Furthermore, the shape of the skull can cause both communicating and noncommunicating hydrocephalus.

Spalding's sign describes overlapping skull bones seen with fetal demise. The bone collapse results from autolysis. This is demonstrated in Figure C of a fetal demise.

Notes

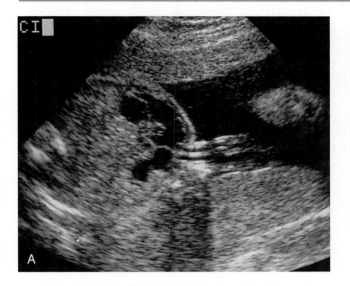
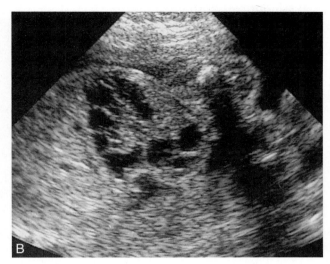

1. Which cystic abnormalities are shown in these axial abdominal images of a mid–second-trimester fetus (Figs. A and B)?

2. How is small bowel obstruction defined?

3. What is the differential diagnosis of dilated fetal small bowel?

4. How does one distinguish large from small bowel obstruction?

Small Bowel (Jejunoileal) Obstruction

1. Dilated small bowel.

2. Persistent loops that are greater than 7 mm in diameter and greater than 15 mm in length.

3. Bowel atresia and stenosis, volvulus, Ladd's bands, and meconium ileus.

4. The ascending and descending colon are peripherally located and show no evidence of peristalsis. Although some of the dilated loops of obstructed small bowel may appear to be peripheral, most will not, and commonly peristalsis is present.

References

Corteville JE, Gray DL, Langer JC: Obstetrics: Bowel abnormalities in the fetus: Correlation of prenatal ultrasonographic findings with outcome. *Am J Obstet Gynecol* 175:724–729, 1996.

Hertzberg BS: Sonography of the fetal gastrointestinal tract: Anatomic variants, diagnostic pitfalls and abnormalities. *AJR Am J Roentgenol* 162:1175–1182, 1994.

Cross-Reference

Ultrasound: THE REQUISITES, pp 258–262.

Comment

Small bowel obstruction occurs in the jejunum and ileum combined as frequently as it does in the duodenum. The incidence of jejunal obstruction is equal to ileal obstruction, with the latter being more commonly distal. Small bowel atresia is the most common cause of fetal small bowel obstruction. Atresia can occur in multiple sites and results from in utero vascular compromise. Cystic fibrosis accounts for 18% to 36% of cases of obstruction.

A large prospective series showed that ultrasound is more sensitive for the prenatal detection of small bowel obstruction than large bowel obstruction. Overall, the diagnosis of small bowel obstruction is made in utero less than 50% of the time. Ultrasound may demonstrate dilatation of small bowel loops, which should not measure more than 7 mm in diameter and 15 mm in length (see Figs. A to D). Other findings include an unusual bowel pattern, ascites (which may be the only finding), polyhydramnios (more common with high obstructions and after 24 weeks), or a cystic abdominal mass (dilated bowel loop as shown earlier). Hyperperistalsis suggests that this cystic mass is small bowel. Whereas a dilated colon is usually peripheral, obstructed small bowel can appear to be partially peripheral as shown in Figures C and D demonstrating a jejunal obstruction.

Fetuses with cystic fibrosis may develop meconium ileus (an ileus owing to thick meconium). This usually

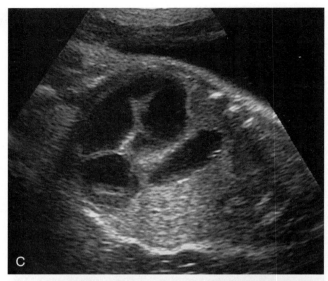

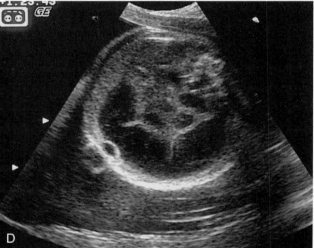

obstructs the ileum and causes proximal small bowel dilatation. It may be accompanied by echogenic bowel and polyhydramnios.

Meconium peritonitis occurs from perforation of the small bowel. Although it may result from bowel obstruction due to cystic fibrosis, it is more commonly associated with small bowel atresia and secondary perforation. Complications of meconium peritonitis include meconium pseudocyst formation which is in the differential diagnosis of a cystic abdominal or pelvic mass. Ascites, typically complicated, and calcification also occur.

Notes

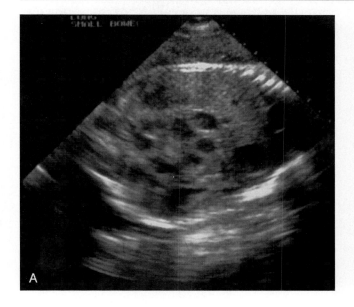

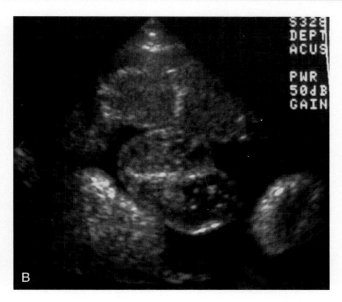

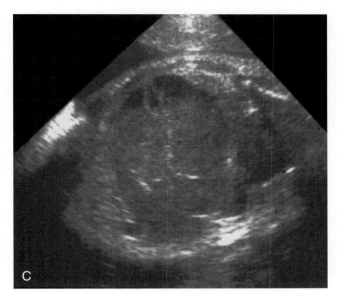

1. What is shown in Figure A (coronal abdomen), Figure B (axial scrotum), and Figure C (axial mid-abdomen)?

2. What is the most common etiology of these findings?

3. What is the most common cause of meconium peritonitis?

4. What is the significance of peritoneal calcifications?

Cystic Fibrosis

1. Figure A—dilated, obstructed small bowel; Figure B—complex scrotal ascites; Figure C—meconium pseudocyst.

2. Meconium peritonitis due to a small bowel perforation.

3. Small bowel atresia.

4. Reflects perforation of bowel and meconium peritonitis in a patient *without* cystic fibrosis (CF).

References

Foster MA, Nyberg DA, Mahoney BS, et al: Meconium peritonitis: Prenatal sonographic findings and their clinical significance. *Radiology* 165:661–665, 1987.

Rypens FF, Avni EF, Abehserva MM, et al: Areas of increased echogenicity in the fetal abdomen: Diagnosis and significance. *Radiographics* 15:1329–1344, 1995.

Cross-Reference

Ultrasound: THE REQUISITES, pp 262–265.

Comment

CF most commonly initially presents with gastrointestinal abnormalities. The enzyme deficiencies of the exocrine glands result in thickened meconium which can obstruct the small bowel or colon. The most common gastrointestinal disorder in CF is meconium ileus, an obstruction of the small bowel with meconium. Occasionally, the abnormality is in the large bowel. Although meconium ileus occurs in only 10% to 15% of infants with CF, almost all cases of meconium ileus result from CF.

On prenatal ultrasound, the small bowel in CF may appear to have an increased echogenicity, although this is not present in approximately 40% of cases. In addition, increased bowel echogenicity is not specific to CF, as it can be a sign of chromosomal anomalies. Obstruction of the small bowel by meconium may be detected as locally dilated bowel. This is usually seen after 26 weeks. Polyhydramnios may be present.

Meconium peritonitis results when an obstructed bowel perforates. Findings on prenatal sonograms include fetal ascites, which is usually complex and echogenic, intra-abdominal calcifications (linear or clumped), bowel dilatation, and polyhydramnios. The differential diagnosis in a newborn includes several etiologies, such as small bowel atresia, meconium ileus, volvulus, internal hernia, intussusception, or congenital band. The presence of peritoneal calcifications reflects an etiology other than CF, because the enzyme deficiency in CF prevents calcification.

The incidence of CF has been reported from 15% to 40% in cases of meconium peritonitis. However, a study by Foster and associates demonstrated that a large percentage of cases of meconium peritonitis detected prenatally with ultrasound are due to other etiologies, including small bowel atresia, stenosis, or volvulus.

Notes

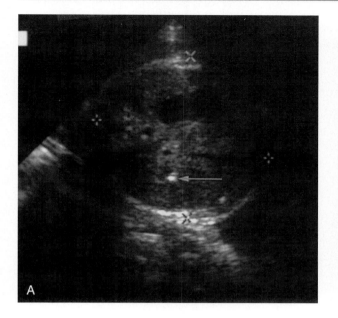

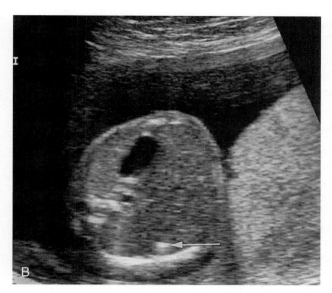

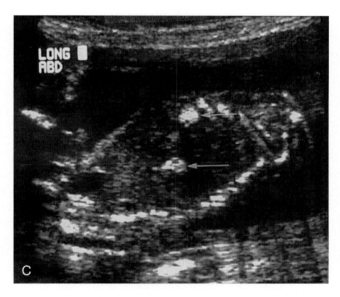

1. Three fetal upper abdominal second-trimester studies (Figs. A and B [axial] and Fig. C [sagittal]) are shown. What do the arrows identify in these cases?

2. What is the cause of fetal intrahepatic calcification?

3. What neonatal liver tumor(s) might contain calcification?

4. What actions should be taken when fetal hepatic calcification is detected?

Fetal Liver Calcifications

1. Figures A and B show intrahepatic calcification. Figure C shows perihepatic calcification.

2. Differential diagnoses include idiopathic, ischemic hepatic necrosis, intrauterine infection, neoplasm if associated with a mass, and rarely portal vein calcification.

3. Hepatoblastoma and metastatic neuroblastoma.

4. Exclude other anomalies and TORCH (toxoplasmosis, other infections, rubella, cytomegalovirus infection, and herpes simplex) infection; follow-up scans.

Reference
Stein B, Bromley B, Michlewitz H, et al: Fetal liver calcifications: Sonographic appearance and postnatal outcome. *Radiology* 197:489–492, 1995.

Cross-Reference
Ultrasound: THE REQUISITES, pp 253–257.

Comment
Hepatic calcifications can arise from various etiologies (see Figs. A and B). These include ischemic hepatic necrosis, intrauterine infection such as cytomegalic virus and toxoplasmosis, a hepatic mass, or rarely calcification in the portal vein. There has been a report of an association with trisomy 9. Perihepatic calcification (see Fig. C) can be seen with meconium peritonitis.

Detection of hepatic calcification warrants a careful search for associated anomalies. A wide spectrum of associated abnormalities have been reported, including intrauterine growth restriction, Hirschsprung's disease, cardiac anomalies, stippled epiphysis, sacral agenesis, and Dandy-Walker variant.

If calcification is an isolated finding, intrauterine infection must be excluded clinically. Follow-up ultrasound studies should be performed. The outcome is good if calcification is an isolated finding, and intrauterine infection is not the cause.

Notes

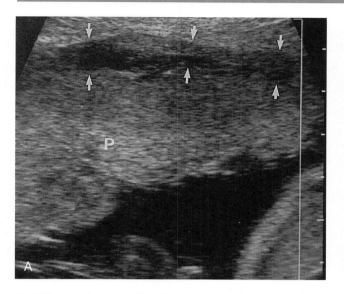

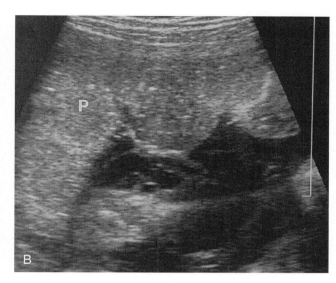

1. Which abnormality (arrows) is shown in this prenatal sonogram of a third-trimester pregnancy (Fig. A; P = placenta)?

2. Figures A and B were obtained at the same time; explain the difference.

3. How do most women present?

4. What is the incidence of fetal death from this condition?

Placental Abruption

1. Placental abruption (retroplacental bleed).

2. The near-gain is normal in Figure A and is set too high in Figure B.

3. Pain or bleeding.

4. 20% to 35% perinatal mortality.

References

Eastman NJ, Hellman LM (eds): *Williams Obstetrics*, 13th ed. Stamford, CT, Appleton-Century-Crofts, 1966, pp 625–632.

Nyberg DA, Cyr DR, Mack LA, et al: Sonographic spectrum of placental abruption. *AJR Am J Roentgenol* 148:161–164, 1987.

Cross-Reference

Ultrasound: THE REQUISITES, pp 317–320.

Comment

Hemorrhage around the placenta is classified according to the location. Many hemorrhages occur in a subchorionic location. Hemorrhage can be located between the placenta and the uterine wall, called retroplacental. If the hemorrhage extends from the retroplacental region lateral to the placenta, it is called marginal. Intraplacental hemorrhage may accompany a retroplacental bleed. A retroplacental hemorrhage that separates the placenta from the uterine wall is called an abruption, which can be partial or complete.

Placental abruption often presents with pelvic/uterine pain and bleeding. The fetal prognosis relates to the volume of hemorrhage and degree of placental separation. The bleed, even if extensive, can decompress if vaginal bleeding is present. If the hemorrhage remains confined to the retroplacental region ("concealed"), the outcome can be worse for the fetus and the mother. This may result in complete placental separation and fetal death, as well as a consumptive coagulopathy in the mother. Risk factors for developing an abruption include maternal hypertension, cigarette smoking, alcohol consumption, cocaine use, trauma, and premature rupture of the membranes.

Ultrasound can demonstrate many of these hemorrhages; a hypoechoic or hyperechoic (depending on the stage) retroplacental collection will be seen, elevating the placenta from the uterine wall. However, if the bleed is entirely isoechoic to placenta, it may not be apparent. This case demonstrates the importance of technique when investigating for an abruption. Figure B fails to identify the abruption seen in Figure A because increased gain falsely fills in the area with echoes. Once an abruption is diagnosed, an assessment of fetal well-being and follow-up ultrasound imaging are important.

Notes

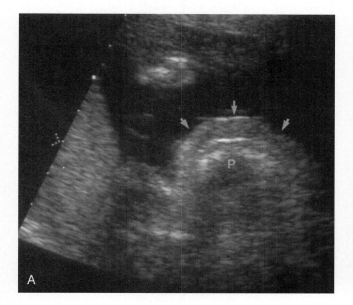

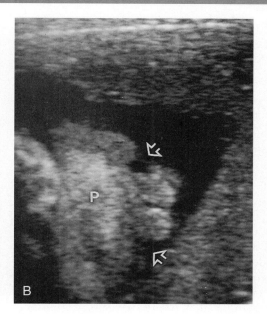

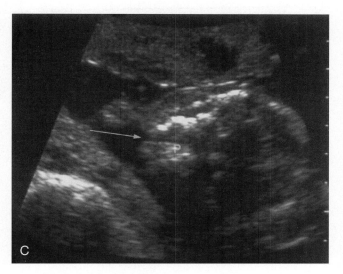

1. Fetus A (Fig. A) shows a normal upper lip (small arrows) and hard palate (P). What are the facial abnormalities identified by the open arrows in fetus B (Fig. B) and by the long arrow in fetus C (Fig. C)? P = hard palate.

2. Name a facial abnormality that may be associated with a bilateral anomaly.

3. What is the ultrasound classification of the spectrum of this anomaly?

4. Does the classification correlate with the outcome?

Cleft Lip and Palate

1. Fetus B has a bilateral cleft lip. Fetus C has a midline cleft lip and palate.

2. Premaxillary protrusion.

3. Type 1: Cleft lip alone; type 2: unilateral cleft lip and palate; type 3: bilateral cleft lip and palate; type 4: midline cleft lip and palate; and type 5: facial defects associated with amniotic bands or limb-body-wall complex.

4. Yes, types 4 and 5 are associated with other anomalies and a fatal outcome.

References

Babcook CJ, McGahan JP, Chong BW, et al: Evaluation of fetal midface anatomy related to facial clefts: Use of US. *Radiology* 201:113–118, 1996.

Nyberg DA, Sickler GK, Hegge FN, et al: Fetal cleft lip with and without cleft palate: US classification and correlation with outcome. *Radiology* 195:677–684, 1995.

Cross-Reference

Ultrasound: THE REQUISITES, pp 215–217.

Comment

Cleft lip is the most common facial anomaly and is associated with cleft palate in 80% of cases. Isolated cleft lip has a better prognosis. When it occurs unilaterally, with or without a cleft palate, it is more commonly seen on the left side. In the setting of bilateral cleft lip and palate, a premaxillary protrusion may be present and was detected in 85% of one series. This soft tissue mass arising from the upper lip occurs when the maxilla is anteriorly displaced.

Nyberg described an ultrasound classification for cleft lip and palate:

Type 1: Cleft lip alone.

Type 2: Unilateral cleft lip and palate.

Type 3: Bilateral cleft lip and palate.

Type 4: Midline cleft lip and palate (see Fig. C).

Type 5: Facial defects associated with amniotic bands or a limb-body-wall complex.

Type 4 and 5 were associated with higher mortality. The poor prognosis of type 4 clefts relates to concurrent anomalies or trisomies, particularly trisomy 13. Type 5 clefts have associated defects of the torso, limb, or cranium as part of the limb-body-wall complex.

Although an evaluation of the palate is not part of the standard prenatal ultrasound scans, it is important because ultrasound can reliably demonstrate the normal facial structures of the lip and hard palate in axial and coronal planes and exclude most cases of cleft lip and palate. Detection of hard palate anomalies is more reli-able before 24 weeks of gestation. Small type 1 and 2 defects may be missed, particularly with a sagittal view. Soft palate abnormalities, when isolated, may also escape detection.

Notes

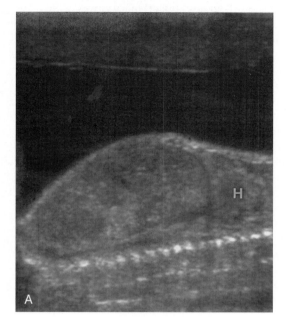

1. What are the two abnormal findings identified in this early third-trimester fetal examination (Fig. A, sagittal image of the left side of fetus; H = heart)?

2. What is the differential diagnosis of absence of the fetal stomach?

3. Does polyhydramnios help to distinguish the etiology?

4. Does gastric nonvisualization occur in all cases of esophageal atresia?

Esophageal Atresia

1. Absence of the fetal stomach and polyhydramnios.

2. Esophageal atresia, congenital diaphragmatic hernia, oligohydramnios, situs abnormality, and impaired swallowing (i.e., central nervous system abnormality, facial cleft, neuromuscular disorder, neck/chest mass, narrow chest).

3. No; it is seen with many of these conditions.

4. No; the stomach may be very small and unchanging.

References

Hertzberg BS: Sonography of the fetal gastrointestinal tract: Anatomic variants, diagnostic pitfalls and abnormalities. *AJR Am J Roentgenol* 162:1175–1182, 1994.

McKenna KM, Goldstein RV, Stringer MD: Small or absent fetal stomach: Prognostic significance. *Radiology* 197:729–733, 1995.

Cross-Reference

Ultrasound: THE REQUISITES, pp 257–259.

Comment

The fetal stomach is seen as a fluid-filled structure in the left upper quadrant by 14 or 15 weeks (and often earlier) in almost all fetuses. Most observers feel that the stomach should always be identified by 19 weeks. Occasionally, nonvisualization of the stomach is a transient normal finding, due to physiologic emptying of the stomach. Rescanning serially over 60 minutes or re-examining at a later date will be expected to demonstrate a fluid-filled stomach in normal cases.

Absence of the fetal stomach or persistently small fetal stomach (<1 cm in size), which persists in the second or third trimester, carries a poor prognosis because of associated conditions. Swallowing dysfunction can be caused by a facial cleft, central nervous system or neuromuscular disorders, a neck/thoracic mass, or a narrow chest due to skeletal dysplasia. The stomach may be located in the thorax (diaphragmatic hernia) or right abdomen (situs abnormality). In true nonvisualization of the stomach, oligohydramnios may be the cause due to decreased amniotic fluid for the fetus to swallow.

Esophageal atresia is often accompanied by nonvisualization of the fetal stomach. However, in some fetuses with a tracheoesophageal fistula, and rarely in those with isolated esophageal atresia, fluid may cross the fistula or gastric secretions may accumulate and minimally distend the stomach (<1 cm in size). In these cases, the stomach will not become more prominent.

Only 50% of fetuses with esophageal atresia are detected in utero either by nonvisualization of the stomach or by polyhydramnios; both are seen in this case (see Fig. A). When seen, they are more commonly identified after 24 weeks. The late onset of findings is a little puzzling and may be due to the failure on the part of the examiner to appreciate a very small stomach as potentially abnormal earlier in the pregnancy and the slow accumulation of amniotic fluid that may not increase above normal until later in the pregnancy. Nevertheless, the presence of polyhydramnios or oligohydramnios with nonvisualization of the stomach has a worse prognosis. Karyotype abnormalities are also associated, including trisomies 18 and 21.

Detection of a small fetal stomach or persistent nonvisualization of the stomach necessitates a careful evaluation for associated anomalies. The mortality depends on the presence or absence of associated abnormalities; the incidence is very high in cases of esophageal atresia because it is part of the VACTERL (*v*ertebral, *a*nal, *c*ardiac, *t*racheoesophageal, *r*enal, and *l*imb) syndrome. The prognosis is better if no other anomalies are associated and the amniotic fluid volume is normal, where in one series 96% of the cases survived.

Notes

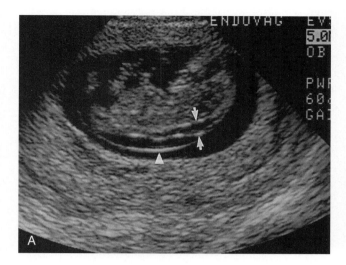

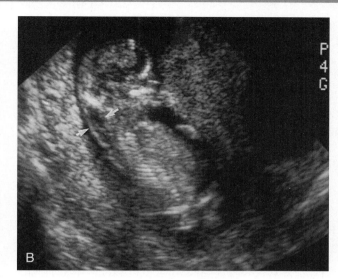

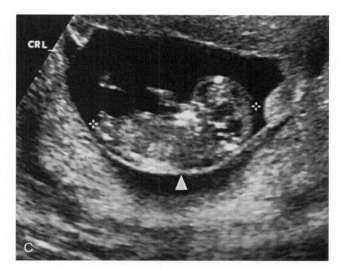

1. Which of these late first-trimester embryos/fetuses (Figs. A to C) are abnormal and why (see *small arrows*)?

2. What is the significance of a septated nuchal lucency?

3. What chromosomal anomalies have been associated with nuchal lucencies?

4. What serum tests are now being combined with nuchal translucency measurements to yield a first-trimester screening tool for chromosomal anomalies?

Nuchal Skin Measurement—First Trimester

1. Figures A and B. Increased nuchal translucency. Arrowheads in Figures A and C point to normal amnion.

2. Septated nuchal lucency has a higher risk of chromosomal abnormality.

3. Trisomies 13, 18, 21, Turner's syndrome (XO), XXX and translocations.

4. Maternal serum free β-human chorionic gonadotropin (HCG) and pregnancy-associated plasma protein A.

References

Spencer K, Souter V, Tul N, et al: A screening program for trisomy 21 at 10–14 weeks using fetal nuchal translucency, maternal serum free beta-human chorionic gonadotropin and pregnancy-associated plasma protein-A. *Ultrasound Obstet Gynecol* 13:231–237, 1999.

Taipale P, Hiilesmaa V, Salonen R, Ylostalo P: Increased nuchal translucency as marker for fetal chromosomal defects. *N Engl J Med* 337:1654–1658, 1997.

van Vugt JMG, Van Zalen-Sprock R, Kostense PJ: First-trimester nuchal translucency: A risk analysis on fetal chromosome abnormality. *Radiology* 200:537–540, 1996.

Cross-Reference
Ultrasound: THE REQUISITES, pp 219–221.

Comment
The nuchal region of the embryo/fetus refers to the soft tissue posterior to the cervical spine or occipital bone. Increased nuchal thickening or translucency are associated with chromosomal anomalies, most commonly Down syndrome, but also trisomies 13 and 18, Turner's syndrome, and translocations.

In the first and early second trimester, the nuchal translucency is usually measured in the sagittal plane, either transabdominally or transvaginally. A translucency thickness of more than 3 mm from 10 to 14 weeks' gestation is considered abnormal. This measurement should include only the anechoic region between two hyperechoic (echogenic) lines. Figures A and B show increased nuchal translucency in two first-trimester fetuses with Down syndrome. It is important to realize that this finding may be limited to this very narrow gestational window. After 14 weeks, the finding may resolve, yet the risk for a chromosomal abnormality remains increased.

At the present time, screening for chromosomal anomalies is performed with a maternal serum triple screen between 15 and 20 weeks. This includes analysis of maternal β-HCG, estriol, and α-fetoprotein. This test alone has only 60% sensitivity for Down syndrome (slightly higher when maternal age is considered), with a high false-positive rate leading to amniocentesis of normal pregnancies. Research is focusing on a new first-trimester screening test. This includes maternal serum free β-HCG and pregnancy-associated plasma protein A as well as a measurement of the nuchal translucency and consideration of maternal age. Studies have shown that a combination of the nuchal translucency and serum markers like these results in a sensitivity of 80% to 90% for detecting Down syndrome, with a 5% false-positive rate.

Notes

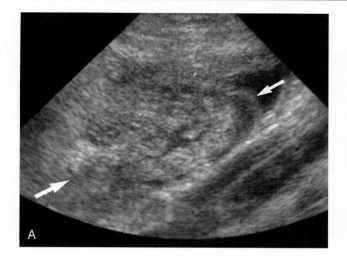

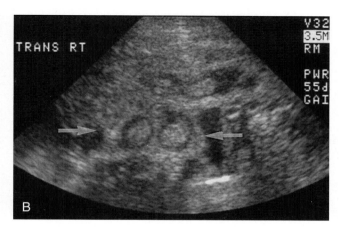

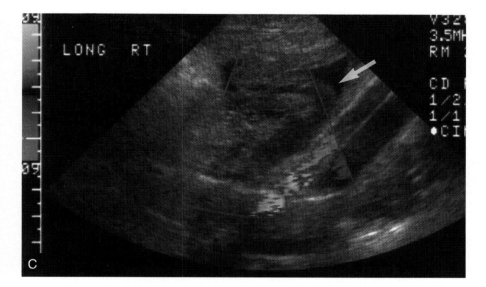

1. An ultrasound examination of the right lower quadrant was performed in a woman 3 days postpartum because of pain (Fig. A [sagittal] and Fig. B [axial] *adjacent to* the right ovary). What do the arrows show? Does the color Doppler image, taken in the same projection as Figure A, confirm your suspicion (Fig. C)? What is your diagnosis?

2. On which side does ovarian vein thrombosis usually occur?

3. What predisposes a woman to ovarian vein thrombosis?

4. Can pulmonary embolism complicate ovarian vein thrombosis?

C A S E 7 6

Ovarian Vein Thrombosis

1. Dilated vein filled with thrombus. Yes. Ovarian vein thrombosis.

2. Right side.

3. Ovarian vein thrombosis can occur after an ectopic pregnancy, abortion, or full-term delivery.

4. Yes.

Acknowledgment

Figures for Case 76 courtesy of Mary C. Frates, MD, and Carol B. Benson, MD, Harvard Medical School, Brigham and Women's Hospital, Boston, MA.

References

Dunnihoo DR, Gallaspy JW, Wise RB, Otterson WN: Postpartum ovarian vein thrombophlebitis: A review. *Obstet Gynecol Surv* 46:415–427, 1991.

Martin B, Mulopulos GP, Bryan PJ: MRI of puerperal ovarian-vein thrombosis (Case Report). *AJR Am J Roentgenol* 147:291–292, 1986.

Cross-Reference

Ultrasound: THE REQUISITES, p 372.

Comment

Ovarian vein thrombosis is caused by an ascending infection following an ectopic pregnancy, abortion, vaginal delivery, or cesarean section. Patients usually present in the first week postpartum with fever, lower abdominal pain, or a tender mass. The right ovarian vein is thrombosed in most cases (80%), both veins in 15%, with isolated left ovarian vein thrombus occurring in only 6% of cases. The differential diagnosis includes other right lower quadrant pathologies: appendicitis, tubo-ovarian abscess, pyelonephritis, ovarian torsion, endometritis, and hematoma of the broad ligament.

Cross-sectional imaging modalities can often confirm the diagnosis. Because the ovarian vein cannot be consistently identified by ultrasound, it is the least reliable. However, when detected, a thrombus of the ovarian vein has the typical appearance of a thrombus elsewhere (see Figs. A and B, arrows). The signs include a hypoechoic or heterogeneous thrombus (depending on its age) distending the vein with pain directly over the region. The distended vein can appear mass-like. The two tubular spaces behind the thrombosed vein (see Fig. A), shown in red and blue on the color Doppler image (see Fig. C), are the normal deeper positioned iliac artery and vein.

Knowledge of the anatomic position of the right ovarian vein, its oblique course adjacent and lateral to the psoas muscle, and its insertion into the inferior vena cava 4 cm below to the right renal vein origin, helps to improve its identification. Color Doppler has been found helpful in evaluating the ovarian vein, inferior vena cava, and renal vein for thrombus propagation (see Fig. C). Enlargement of the ipsilateral ovary is an important secondary finding.

Magnetic resonance imaging (MRI) is accurate in detecting ovarian vein thrombosis, and a single case report suggests that MRI can differentiate acute from subacute thrombus, using the signal intensity of the clot.

Complications of ovarian vein thrombosis include right-sided hydronephrosis, pulmonary or septic emboli, Budd-Chiari syndrome, and hepatic infarction as well as renal vein or inferior vena cava thrombosis.

Notes

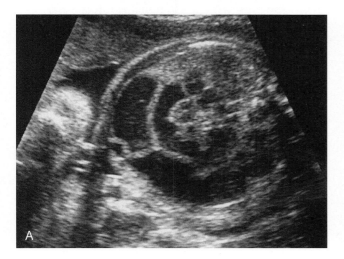

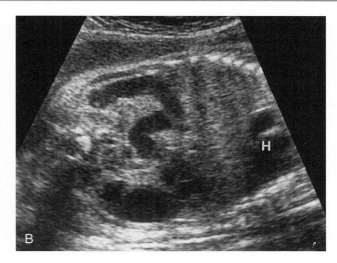

1. In this third-trimester fetus, what is the likely anatomic location of this bowel obstruction (Fig. A is an axial image of the mid fetal abdomen; Fig. B is a coronal image of the fetal body. H = heart)?

2. What is the differential diagnosis of a dilated fetal colon?

3. Would sacral agenesis aid in distinguishing the possible etiologies?

4. At what gestational age is colon dilatation due to anorectal atresia more likely to be diagnosed on prenatal ultrasound?

Large Bowel (Anorectal) Atresia

1. Distal colon.

2. Anorectal atresia, Hirschsprung's disease, and meconium plug syndrome.

3. Yes.

4. After 27 weeks.

Reference
Harris RD, Nyberg DA, Mack LA, Weinberger E: Anorectal atresia: Prenatal sonographic diagnosis. *AJR Am J Roentgenol* 149:395–400, 1987.

Cross-Reference
Ultrasound: THE REQUISITES, pp 258–262.

Comment
Anorectal atresia is often one manifestation of a spectrum of anomalies as part of the VACTERL syndrome, which includes vertebral, anorectal, cardiovascular, tracheo-esophageal, renal, and limb anomalies. In neonates, almost 75% of cases will have such associated malformations. Anorectal atresia can also be seen as part of the caudal regression syndrome. A careful search for associated anomalies is imperative as one ultrasound series demonstrated other VACTERL anomalies in more than 90% of the fetuses with anorectal atresia. The differential diagnosis of dilated colon includes Hirschsprung's disease, anorectal atresia, and meconium plug syndrome; the latter two are associated with maternal diabetes.

The fetal bowel normally becomes more dilated with increasing gestational age. Normal fetuses have a mean colon diameter of 15 to 16 mm at term, and the upper limits of normal approach 20 mm. In anorectal atresia, the bowel dilatation is often greater than 2 standard deviations (SDs) above the mean for any given gestational age. A dilated colon is often peripheral in location (see Figs. A and B); however, some cases of small bowel dilatation can appear peripheral. Tracing the dilatation to the rectosigmoid colon in the pelvis (see Fig. B) aids in confirming that the obstructed bowel is colon. Peristalsis has been described in dilated large bowel loops but would be considered unusual (dilated small bowel loops more commonly show peristalsis).

One series stated that prenatal ultrasound detects less than 10% of cases of large bowel obstruction. The presence of dilated bowel in anorectal atresia correlates with the gestational age. The bowel does not dilate before 22 weeks but will often show progressive dilatation and can be detected after 27 weeks. The presence of a perineal fistula does not correlate with degree of bowel dilatation. Oligohydramnios and occasionally polyhydramnios have been reported, both likely related to the commonly present additional abnormalities.

Notes

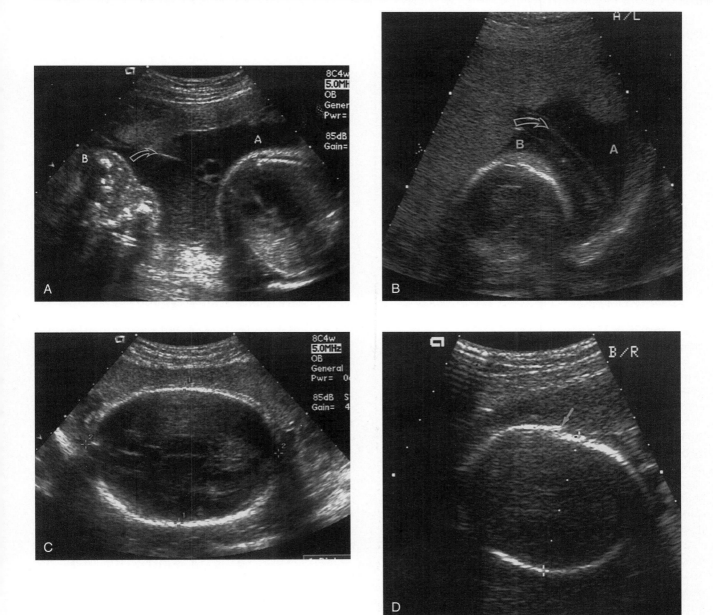

1. A woman with a known twin pregnancy presents at 24 weeks for a routine assessment of twin growth. Figures A and B show both fetuses (fetus A on the reader's right and fetus B on the reader's left) and the separating membrane (open arrow). Is this a dichorionic or monochorionic pregnancy and why?

2. Additional images of the fetal heads, Figure C (fetus A) and Figure D (fetus B). The arrow in Figure D denotes a calvarial suture line. What is the most likely diagnosis and why?

3. If there is fetal demise in a twin gestation, what trimester is most likely?

4. If one of the twins dies in a dichorionic pregnancy, is there increased risk of demise for the other fetus?

Second-Trimester Twin Gestation and Fetal Demise

1. Dichorionic pregnancy. The intervening membrane is well defined and more than 2 mm in thickness.

2. Demise of fetus B. Fetus B shows overlapping of calvarial sutures (see Fig. D, arrow) with poorly defined internal anatomy. Amniotic fluid surrounding fetus B appears decreased.

3. The first trimester.

4. Little to none. If the demise occurs late in the second and third trimester, labor can infrequently be induced, or the demised fetus may obstruct the delivery of the normal fetus.

Reference

Richard JA, MacDonald PC, Gant F (eds): *Williams Obstetrics,* 17th ed. Norwalk, CT, Appleton-Century-Crofts, 1985, pp 212–217.

Cross-Reference

Ultrasound: THE REQUISITES, p 351.

Comment

In 80% of cases, twin gestations occur in their own separate sacs (dichorionic-diamniotic [Di-Di]) and, therefore, have separate environments. In the other 20%, the twins develop within the same monochorionic environment, either partially or completely. They then partially share the same environment and are diamniotic (monochorionic-dichorionic [Mono-Di]) or completely share the same environment and are monoamniotic (Mono-Mono), both with intermingled placental circulations.

The rate of spontaneous abortion (miscarriage) in singleton pregnancies is approximately 20% to 25%. This rate is slightly higher in twin gestations. In a Di-Di pregnancy, a first-trimester loss of one of the twins may not be noticed. If incidentally detected by ultrasound, the demised twin will show either an abnormal empty sac or a sac containing an embryo without heart motion or an abnormal yolk sac. In these cases, if the pregnancies are followed, the demised twin will "vanish" leaving one developing gestational sac. In a monochorionic twinning, because of the shared circulation, the demised twin may adversely affect the living twin.

In the second and third trimester, a spontaneous loss of one of the twins is uncommon. However, even in Di-Di twin pregnancies, the loss rate is slightly higher than in singleton pregnancies, partially due to the somewhat higher incidence for growth restriction. With monochorionic pregnancies, there are additional problems because of the shared placental circulation, which could lead to a twin-twin transfusion; late in the pregnancy if the pregnancy is monoamniotic, there is also the potential complication of demise due to entangled umbilical cords.

When there is a loss of a twin in a Di-Di pregnancy in the second or third trimester, the demise should not adversely affect the living fetus (see Figs. A to D). The demised fetus will, of course, have no detectable heart motion. Because autolysis occurs within the first week, the demised fetus will lose its internal anatomy and will begin to collapse. The fetal head of the demised fetus B (see Fig. D) shows no demonstrable internal anatomy and overlapping of calvarial sutures (arrow), called the Spaulding sign. Additionally, there appears to be a decrease in the amount of amniotic fluid in the sac surrounding fetus B (see Figs. A and B), a finding also noted in fetal demise. The increased echogenicity of the fluid, however, is of uncertain significance.

The diagnosis of dichorionic pregnancy is important, because it helps predict the risk to the remaining fetus. This can be determined by the following: different fetal genders, separate placentas, or a thick, well-defined membrane. The membrane is better defined in the first trimester, but when clearly seen in the second or third trimester it is indicative of a dichorionic pregnancy (see Figs. A and B).

The demised twin in the second and third trimester will not "vanish." Instead, in a Di-Di pregnancy, the fetus may flatten and be pushed to one side but may still be visible even at term. This is called a fetus papraceous (paper fetus). This fetus, although not directly impinging on the other fetus, may cause either spontaneous labor or, at term, may block the exit of the normal fetus. If the pregnancy is monochorionic, the shared placental circulation may create significant problems for the living remaining fetus, most likely owing to disseminated intravascular coagulopathy. This can cause in utero demise or destruction (embolic) changes in the surviving fetus.

Notes

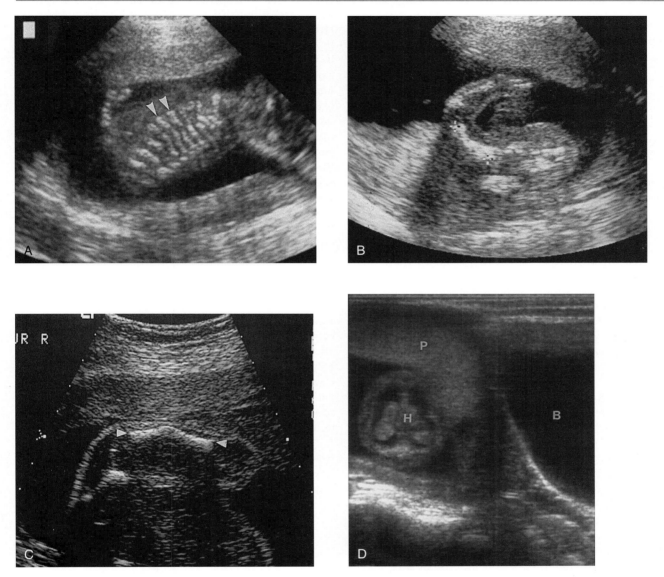

1. In this 22-week-old fetus (fetus A), which abnormalities are detected in the sagittal image of the fetal chest (Fig. A, arrows) and long axis image of one of the femurs (Fig. B; +'s = femoral shaft)? What is your most likely diagnosis, and what is the level of severity?

2. In another fetus (fetus B) at 35 weeks of age with the same disorder, what is seen in this image of one of its femurs (Fig. C; arrowheads = the femoral shaft)? If this is the only bone involved, is this case likely to be as severe as in the case of fetus A?

3. Can osteogenesis imperfecta (OI) be ruled out by a normal ultrasound examination?

4. What is the underlying biochemical abnormality in OI?

Osteogenesis Imperfecta

1. Rib fracture and bowed femur with grossly normal bone brightness. Osteogenesis imperfecta—severe.

2. Angled bone due to a healed fracture with normal bone brightness. No, less severe.

3. No.

4. OI is a connective tissue disorder with defective type I collagen.

Acknowledgment

Figures A and B for Case 79 courtesy of Beryl Benacerraf, MD.

References

Bulas DI, Stern HJ, Rosenbaum KN, et al: Variable prenatal appearance of osteogenesis imperfecta. *J Ultrasound Med* 13:419–427, 1994.

Munoz C, Filly RA, Golbus MS: Osteogenesis imperfecta type II: Prenatal sonographic diagnosis. *Radiology* 174:181–185, 1990.

Pretorius DH, Rumack CM, Manc-Johnson ML, et al: Specific skeletal dysplasias in utero: Sonographic diagnosis. *Radiology* 159:237–242, 1986.

Cross-Reference

Ultrasound: THE REQUISITES, pp 299–300.

Comment

OI is a connective tissue disorder that is attributed to defective type I collagen. Various organ systems may be involved, including the eyes (sclerae), skin, teeth, and ears; however, the most widely recognized abnormalities involve the skeletal system. The outcome ranges from mild affliction (e.g., osteoporosis) to stillbirth or early neonatal death.

A classification system has been described using genetic, clinical, and radiographic criteria. Types I and IV are autosomal dominant and nonlethal. Type I has mildly fragile bones without significant deformity, whereas type IV presents with osteoporosis and fragile bones that bow. Types II and III are more severe. Type II can be autosomal dominant, wherein most affected fetuses die, and type III presents as nonlethal autosomal recessive. Type II has demineralization and multiple fractures, whereas type III presents with fractures that result in deformed bones and spine.

The ultrasound diagnosis relies on the detection of fractures, unusual bowing of the long bones, and decreased bone brightness. If none of these is present, the diagnosis of OI cannot be made, even in the appropriate clinical and biochemical setting. Therefore, the lack of positive ultrasound findings cannot rule out an affected fetus.

The ultrasound criteria for the lethal type II OI centers not only on marked deformities or fractures but also on bone demineralization, particularly of the calvarium. Demineralization cannot be quantitated but is suggested by the lack of normal bone brightness. This is shown in a third affected fetus, fetus C (Fig. D). Figure D, an axial view of the head (H), shows normal internal anatomy, including the choroid plexuses but no normal calvarial brightness. (P = placenta; B = urinary bladder.) The differential diagnosis of skull demineralization includes congenital hypophosphatasia and achondrogenesis, both of which may have poor ossification of the spine, with less than three ossification centers characteristic of the latter.

Fractures can be multiple and involve long bones and ribs, which may also appear bowed or beaded, as in type III OI (fetus A, see Figs. A and B). A "wrinkled appearance" has been used to describe the femur with multiple fractures. If the spine can be clearly imaged, the vertebral bodies may be flattened, called platyspondyly, caused by softening of the vertebral bodies. Polyhydramnios may be present.

Prenatal diagnosis of the nonlethal subtypes may be more difficult. Bowing or angulation at the point of a fracture may be seen as in fetus B (see Fig. C). Normally, only the inner surface of the femur can appear mildly bowed. Any other long bone with bowing could be considered abnormal. Mineralization, identified on ultrasound as brightness, is usually normal. Limb length can be normal to moderately shortened.

Notes

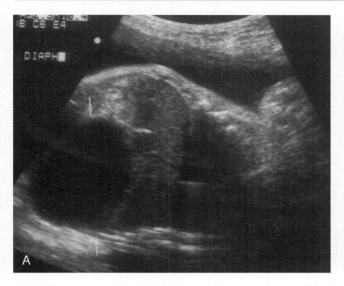

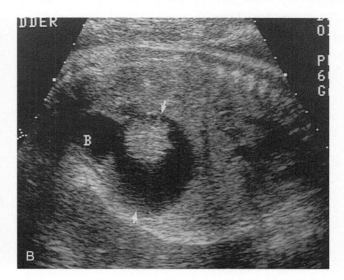

1. What is the most likely origin of the cystic abdominopelvic mass (arrow) shown in the third-trimester female fetus (Fig. A)? What is the cause?

2. Which fetal ovarian mass (arrows) can have cystic and solid components (Fig. B)? B = urinary bladder.

3. What are the potential complications of an ovarian cyst?

4. What endocrine syndrome has been described in association with fetal ovarian cysts?

Fetal Ovarian Cyst

1. Ovarian cyst; maternal hormones crossing the placenta.

2. Teratoma.

3. Rupture, torsion, hemorrhage, bowel obstruction, and dystocia.

4. Congenital hypothyroidism.

References

Crombleholme TM, Craigo SD, Garmel S, D'Alton ME: Fetal ovarian cyst decompression to prevent torsion. *J Pediatr Surg* 32:1447-1449, 1997.

Jafri SZH, Bree RL, Silver TM, Ouimette M: Fetal ovarian cysts: Sonographic detection and association with hypothyroidism. *Radiology* 150:809-812, 1984.

Cross-Reference

Ultrasound: THE REQUISITES, pp 269-271.

Comment

Small follicular ovarian cysts have been detected in one third of stillbirths and neonatal female deaths. Ovarian cysts are usually functional and histologically benign, induced by maternal hormones crossing the placenta. In girls, ovarian cysts occur in association with long-standing hypothyroidism. This is a result of precocious sexual development. The pituitary secretes a nonspecific glycoprotein hormone as a result of hypothyroidism. Fetal ovarian cysts have been detected prenatally on ultrasound in the setting of congenital hypothyroidism.

On ultrasound, a simple ovarian cystic mass (see Fig. A) will be identified in the pelvis if small or extending out of the pelvis into the abdomen if large. Polyhydramnios has been reported in 10% of cases, possibly due to small bowel obstruction by large cysts. Bilateral cysts have been described. Fetal ovarian teratomas (see Fig. B) appear as cystic and solid masses of the ovary.

Complications include hemorrhage and bowel obstruction in addition to ovarian torsion. The cyst can rupture at delivery or cause dystocia due to abdominal distention if it is large.

Decompression has been recommended in the literature from large centers that perform in utero surgery, although this is controversial. It is recommended, however, when the cyst is larger than 4 cm, enlarges rapidly (>1 cm/wk), or can be shown to move around the fetal abdomen on serial ultrasounds. These signs are considered to be indicators of an increased risk of torsion. Fetal ovarian cysts can resolve spontaneously. Ultrasound is performed postnatally, and the cysts can be aspirated in the neonate if necessary.

Notes

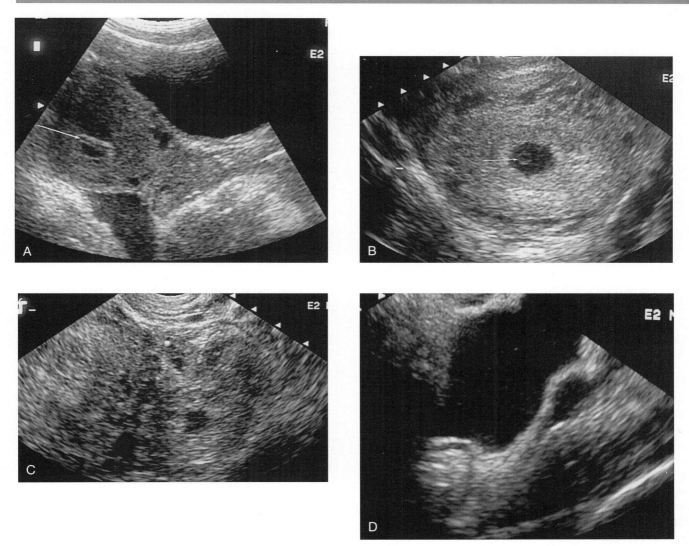

1. What is the diagnosis in this early first-trimester ultrasound examination (Figs. A and B are transabdominal sagittal scans and transvaginal axial scans of the uterus, and Figures C and D are transvaginal axial scans of the right adnexa)?

2. What is the incidence of *spontaneous* heterotopic pregnancy? The incidence has increased in high-risk groups to as high as 1 in 3000. What accounts for the rise?

3. What is the incidence of heterotopic pregnancy after assisted reproduction?

4. What are the treatment options?

Heterotopic Pregnancy

1. Heterotopic pregnancy: concomitant intrauterine and extrauterine pregnancies.

2. 1 in 30,000. Assisted reproduction and pelvic inflammatory disease.

3. Up to 3%.

4. Salpingectomy, salpingostomy, and direct infusion of potassium chloride into the ectopic gestation (salpingocentesis).

References

Rojansky N, Schenker JG: Heterotopic pregnancy and assisted reproduction—an update. *J Assist Reprod Genet* 13:554–601, 1996.

Tal J, Haddad S, Gordon N, Timor-Tritsch I: Heterotopic pregnancy after ovulation induction and assisted reproductive technologies: A literature review from 1971–1993. *Fertil Steril* 66:1–12, 1996.

Cross-Reference
Ultrasound: THE REQUISITES, pp 416, 427.

Comment

The occurrence of an intrauterine pregnancy with a simultaneous extrauterine gestation was once a rare phenomenon, with spontaneous incidence estimated at 1 in 30,000 pregnancies. However, in recent years, several factors have led to an increase in the incidence of heterotopic pregnancy: assisted reproduction techniques (ART), intrauterine contraceptive devices, pelvic inflammatory disease, and previous tubal surgery. In these high-risk groups, the incidence of heterotopic pregnancy has been estimated to be as high as 1 in 3000. For women undergoing ART, this complication occurs in 1% to 3%.

In cases where women have undergone ART, the diagnosis is often made with a screening ultrasound early in the gestation while the woman is asymptomatic. Symptomatic patients present with abdominal pain in most cases, and vaginal bleeding occurs in only 50% (owing to the concomitant intrauterine gestation).

Improvements in ultrasound have resulted in an increased rate of detection for heterotopic pregnancies, particularly using transvaginal imaging. However, a preliminary transabdominal scan is essential to exclude any mass in a suprauterine location or the rare abdominal pregnancy. In a heterotopic pregnancy, in addition to the intrauterine gestation, ultrasound may demonstrate a live extrauterine gestation, an adnexal gestational sac, or an adnexal mass. The case shown here demonstrates an intrauterine pregnancy (see Figs. A and B), with an intrauterine gestational sac in Figure A and a yolk sac in Figure B (arrows). In the right adnexa, a thick-walled cystic mass (see Fig. C), and moderate free cul-de-sac fluid (see Fig. D) were also identified. Although the presence of an intrauterine gestation formerly excluded an ectopic pregnancy, in any woman with risk factors for heterotopic pregnancy, careful evaluation for an adnexal mass or complex fluid must be performed. It is important to keep in mind that a ruptured corpus luteum cyst can also result in a moderate amount of intraperitoneal hemorrhage.

Treatment options are aimed at salvaging the intrauterine pregnancy. Salpingectomy, salpingoscopic removal, and salpingocentesis (direct infusion of potassium chloride into the ectopic gestation) have all been performed. Oophorectomy is performed for the rare ovarian heterotopic pregnancy.

The outcome depends somewhat on the location of the heterotopic pregnancy. Cornual heterotopic pregnancies are particularly hazardous owing to hemoperitoneum, with a lower rate of survival for the intrauterine gestation. Overall, the intrauterine gestation survival rate is 60% to 70%.

Notes

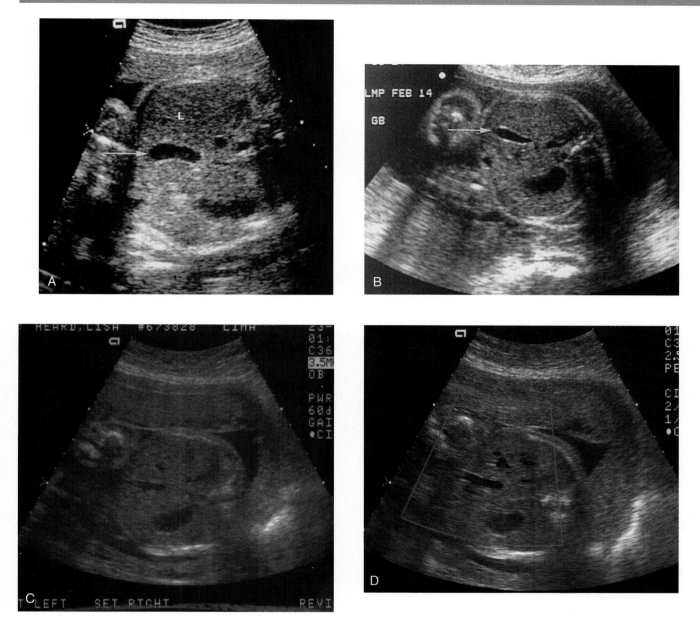

1. What is the most likely diagnosis and the differential diagnosis of the two fluid-filled structures in the upper abdomen of these mid–second-trimester fetuses (Figs. A and B, axial images of the upper abdomen. L = liver)?

2. What fluid-filled upper abdominal structure do these additional images (Figs. C and D) of the upper abdomen detect (same fetus as in Fig. B)?

3. When is the gallbladder usually seen?

4. Does nonvisualization of the fetal gallbladder predict biliary atresia?

Fetal Gallbladder

1. Fetal gallbladder. Differential diagnosis includes a dilated or normal portal (intra-abdominal portion of the umbilical) vein and cystic abdominal masses (e.g., duplication, mesenteric cyst, choledochal).

2. The normal umbilical portion of the left portal vein.

3. Between 24 and 32 weeks.

4. No.

References

Hertzberg BS, Kliewer MA, Bowie JD, et al: Enlarged fetal gallbladder: Prognostic importance for aneuploidy or biliary abnormality at antenatal US. *Radiology* 208:795–798, 1998.

Hertzberg BS, Kliewer MA, Maynor C, et al: Nonvisualization of the fetal gallbladder: Frequency and prognostic importance. *Radiology* 199:679–682, 1996.

Cross-Reference

Ultrasound: THE REQUISITES, pp 253–257.

Comment

The fetal gallbladder can be seen in 80% of prenatal ultrasound studies if careful scanning is performed. It is seen more frequently between 24 and 32 weeks, and visualization declines later in the gestation, perhaps due to gallbladder contractions near term. In fetuses in whom the gallbladder is not visualized, the outcome is usually normal, with no increased incidence of biliary tract anomalies or cystic fibrosis.

The fetal gallbladder enlarges progressively through the gestation. The average area is 8 mm² between 12 and 15 weeks and is as large as 91 mm² between 32 and 35 weeks. "Cholecystomegaly," or gallbladder enlargement, is not associated with biliary tract abnormalities. Infants with trisomy 13 have an increased incidence of gallbladder enlargement; however, this is not a predictor of chromosomal anomalies on prenatal ultrasound.

The gallbladder may extend directly anteriorly (see Figs. A and B) and can be mistaken for the normal umbilical portion of the left portal vein (see Figs. C and D). It should not be mistaken for an umbilical varix, which is a focal dilatation of the intra-abdominal umbilical vein just inside the abdominal wall, which can be distinguished by color Doppler. A prominent gallbladder should not be mistaken for a cystic abdominal mass.

Notes

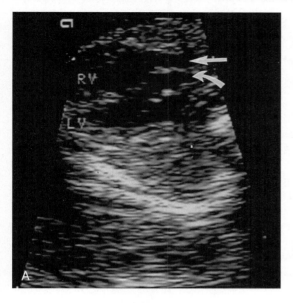

1. What is the abnormality shown in this image of the outflow tracts of the heart (Fig. A; RV = right ventricle; LV = left ventricle)?

2. What is the diagnosis?

3. Which great vessel is anterior in transposition of the great vessels (TGV)?

4. How do the ventricles appear on a four-chamber view in TGV?

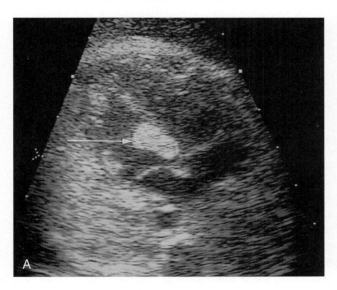
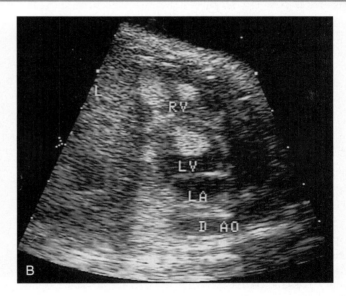

1. Images of a second trimester fetal heart are presented. What is the most common etiology for the intracardiac abnormalities on the axial view (Fig. A, shown by arrow in the left ventricle) and sagittal view (Fig. B) of both ventricles? RV = right ventricle; LV = left ventricle; LA = left atrium; D AO = descending thoracic aorta.

2. What percentage of cardiac rhabdomyomas are associated with tuberous sclerosis?

3. What percentage of patients with tuberous sclerosis have cardiac rhabdomyomas?

4. What percentage of cardiac rhabdomyomas are multiple?

CASE 83

Transposition of the Great Vessels

1. Parallel great vessels.

2. Transposition of the great vessels.

3. Aorta.

4. Most commonly normal.

Acknowledgment
Figure A for Case 83 courtesy of Dennis Wood.

References
Allan LD: Sonographic detection of parallel great arteries in the fetus. *AJR Am J Roentgenol* 168:1283–1286, 1997.

Benacerraf BR: Sonographic detection of fetal anomalies of the aortic and pulmonary arteries: Value of the four-chamber view vs. direct images. *AJR Am J Roentgenol* 163:1483–1489, 1994.

Cross-Reference
Ultrasound: THE REQUISITES, pp 238–243.

Comment
TGV is the most common anomaly of great vessel position. The aorta is located anteriorly and arises from the right ventricle (see Fig. A; straight arrow = aorta). The pulmonary artery arises posteriorly from the left ventricle (see Fig. A; curved arrow = main pulmonary artery). The ventricles are in their normal position in D-TGV, with the aorta on the right of the pulmonary artery. In corrected transposition, or L-TGV, the ventricles are also reversed, so that the aorta is located to the left of the pulmonary artery. Corrected TGV is associated with a number of other cardiac malformations, including ventricular septal defect, arrhythmias, and peripheral pulmonic stenosis, any of which contribute to morbidity.

On the prenatal sonogram, the four-chamber view is usually normal with TGV. Therefore, an evaluation of the outflow tracts is essential. The normal aorta arises posteriorly from the left ventricle and courses right and cranially, then posteriorly. The normal pulmonary artery originates from the anterior right ventricle and runs posteriorly, crossing over the origin of the aorta. A parallel relationship of the proximal aorta to the pulmonary trunk indicates TGV, as shown in this case. One should be aware that *more distally*, the aorta and pulmonary artery may run parallel for a short course.

The differential diagnosis of parallel great vessels is a double-outlet right ventricle. This cardiac anomaly is commonly associated with other systemic malformations.

Notes

CASE 84

Cardiac Rhabdomyoma

1. Intracardiac rhabdomyomas.

2. 50% to 78%.

3. 50% to 60%.

4. 90%.

Acknowledgment
Figures A and B for Case 84 courtesy of Dennis Woods.

References
Paladini D, Palmierie S, Russo MG, Pacileo G: Cardiac multiple rhabdomyomatosis: Prenatal diagnosis and natural history. *Ultrasound Obstet Gynecol* 7:84–85, 1996.

Seki I, Singh AD, Longo S: Pathologic case of the month: Congenital cardiac rhabdomyoma. *Arch Pediatr Adolesc Med* 150:877–878, 1996.

Uzon O, McGawley G, Wharton GA: Multiple cardiac rhabdomyomas: Tuberous sclerosis or not. *Heart* 77:388, 1997.

Cross-Reference
Ultrasound: THE REQUISITES, pp 240–241.

Comment
The most common cardiac mass in the fetus, infant, and child is a rhabdomyoma. Ninety percent are multiple. The differential considerations (fibroma and myxoma) are much less common and occur as isolated masses. Of patients diagnosed with cardiac rhabdomyomas, 50% to 78% have tuberous sclerosis. Conversely, 50% to 60% of patients with tuberous sclerosis have cardiac rhabdomyomas. Tuberous sclerosis is an autosomal dominant syndrome with variable expression.

Cardiac rhabdomyoma can be detected on prenatal ultrasound. Single or multiple, homogeneously hyperechoic masses are seen in the right or left ventricle; the case shown above demonstrates two masses in the right ventricle and one in the left. These arise from the intraventricular septum or ventricular wall. The masses show a biphasic growth in utero, enlarging until 32 weeks' gestational age and subsequently shrinking in the first year of life. If detected, follow-up imaging is required to identify complications of arrhythmia, cardiac failure, and hydrops.

Rhabdomyomas are histologically benign, and small rhabdomyomas that do not cause hemodynamic abnormalities regress in 80% before 4 years of age. Complications of larger masses include intracardiac flow obstruction and arrhythmia. Such sequelae carry a poor prognosis.

Notes

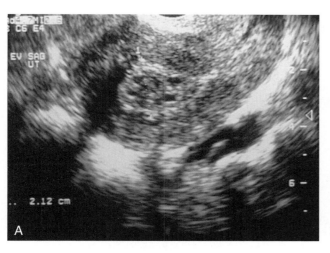
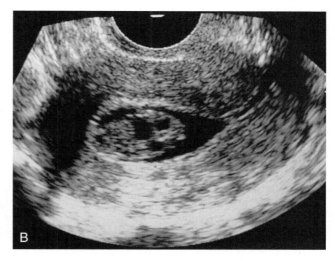

1. This 40-year-old woman presents with vaginal bleeding. A sagittal transvaginal ultrasound of the uterus (Fig. A) shows a focal heterogeneous endometrial thickening of 21 mm (+'s). What are the differential diagnoses, and could any other ultrasound procedure elucidate this problem?

2. A follow-up transvaginal sonohysterogram (SHG) in the same sagittal projection as Figure A was performed (Fig. B). Does this aid in making the diagnosis? If so, what is your diagnosis?

3. What accounts for the cystic (anechoic) spaces in endometrial polyps on ultrasound?

4. What is the typical echogenicity of an endometrial polyp versus a submucosal or intracavitary myoma?

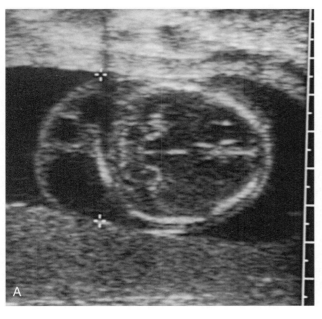
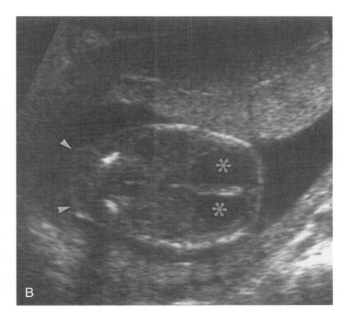

1. What are the diagnoses of the posterior neck masses shown in fetus A (Fig. A; +'s = mass) and fetus B (Fig. B; arrowheads = soft tissue mass)?

2. What findings will aid in distinction?

3. Will the α-fetoprotein (AFP) level aid in distinction?

4. In which entity is karyotype testing warranted?

Endometrial Polyp

1. Polyp, focal hyperplasia, and cancer. A sonohysterogam would better define the abnormality.

2. Yes; a pedunculated polyp.

3. Dilated glands.

4. Hyperechoic; hypoechoic.

Acknowledgement

Figures A & B courtesy of Dr. Anna Lev-Toaff, MD.

References

Hulka CA, Hall DA, McCarthy K, Simeone JF: Endometrial polyps, hyperplasia and carcinoma in postmenopausal women: Differentiation with endovaginal sonography. *Radiology* 191:755–758, 1994.

Lev-Toaff AS, Toaff ME, Liu J-B, et al: Value of sonohysterography in the diagnosis and management of abnormal uterine bleeding. *Radiology* 201:179–184, 1996.

Cross-Reference

Ultrasound: THE REQUISITES, pp 368–374.

Comment

Causes of dysfunctional uterine bleeding include complications of pregnancy, polyp, myoma, endometrial atrophy, hyperplasia, and endometrial cancer.

The appearance of the endometrium has been shown to have some correlation with the pathologic process, although there is overlap in appearances. As shown in this case, polyps are typically hyperechoic and often have small cystic spaces due to dilated glands (see Figs. A and B). Myomata are usually hypoechoic; they absorb sound and can be submucosal or completely intracavitary. Hyperplasia is often uniformly hyperechoic and can demonstrate cystic spaces. A heterogeneous thickened endometrium is a common appearance for endometrial cancer, which has been shown to present with a greater degree of endometrial thickening than the benign causes.

Once a thickened endometrium is diagnosed, dilatation and curettage are often performed. However, due to sampling error, the pathologic diagnosis can be missed, particularly when only a portion of the endometrium appears to be thickened (see Fig. A). In many cases, a sonohysterogram (SHG) is useful (see Fig. B) and in this case confirms the diagnosis of an endome trial polyp. The SHG is performed by instilling sterile saline into the uterine cavity under ultrasound guidance. The information can guide the gynecologist to the site of biopsy. Using an SHG, one can distinguish a polyp (as shown in this case) from a myoma and define the exact location of a myoma (intracavitary versus submucosal versus myometrial), which dictates whether surgery can be performed hysteroscopically. Therefore, many management decisions are aided by the findings on an SHG.

Notes

Posterior Neck Mass

1. Fetus A (see Fig. A) is a cystic hygroma. Fetus B (see Fig. B) is an encephalocele.

2. For cystic hygroma, a "spoke-wheel" appearance of septations is pathognomonic (see Fig. A). For an encephalocele, a cranial defect and central nervous system (CNS) abnormalities are associated.

3. Yes. AFP is usually normal in encephaloceles but can be elevated in a cystic hygroma or cervical meningomyelocele.

4. Both.

Reference

Goldstein RB, LaPidus AS, Filly RA: Fetal cephaloceles: Diagnosis with US. *Radiology* 180:803–808, 1991.

Cross-Reference

Ultrasound: THE REQUISITES, pp 218–219.

Comment

Careful ultrasound evaluation of a posterior neck mass is essential to making an accurate diagnosis.

Cephaloceles, cervical meningomyeloceles, and cystic hygromas can be entirely cystic. Even with an encephalocele, the CNS matter may not be apparent on ultrasound. If solid material or a definite cranial defect (see Fig. B, posterior) is identified, then an encephalocele can be ensured. However, in many cases the cranial defect is difficult to visualize, or a dropout artifact creates a spurious defect. A cyst-within-a-cyst appearance has been described with an encephalocele and may represent a herniated, dilated fourth ventricle into the encephalocele.

The presence of septations (see Fig. A), particularly a "spoke-wheel appearance," suggests a cystic hygroma. Most cephaloceles and cervical meningomyeloceles are midline defects, and cystic hygromas can be posterior or posterolateral. A cephalocele can rarely be caused by an amniotic band syndrome and is almost always asymmetric. Although cephaloceles usually have an acute angle between the mass and the skin line, a cystic hygroma usually creates an obtuse angle with the skin.

The presence of specific associated findings may aid in distinction. CNS abnormalities including ventriculomegaly (see Fig. B), lemon-head deformity, beaked tectum, flattened basioccipital bone, and microcephaly suggest a cephalocele or cervical meningomyelocele. Cystic hygroma can be complicated by serous effusions and subcutaneous edema (hydrops).

Notes

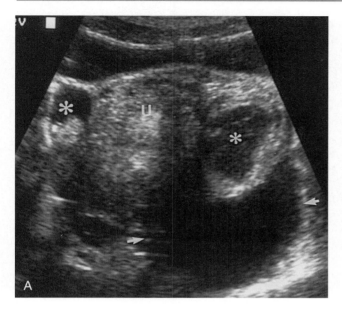

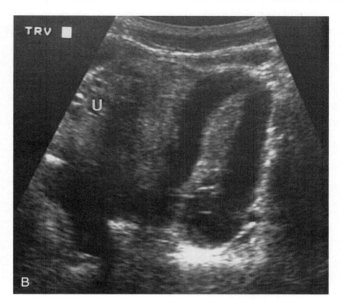

1. A 19-year-old woman presents with pelvic pain and fever. The result of her pregnancy test is negative, and she has a past medical history of treated pelvic infection. What are the findings and most likely diagnosis from the transabdominal ultrasound examination (Figs. A and B)? Figure A is an axial image of the uterus (U) and adnexa (asterisks). Figure B is a slightly higher axial image of the uterus (U) and left adnexa.

2. Is a hydrosalpinx better detected by a transabdominal or transvaginal study?

3. Do clinicians often order an ultrasound examination in cases of pelvic inflammatory disease (PID)?

4. Are patients with PID at a greater risk for an ectopic pregnancy?

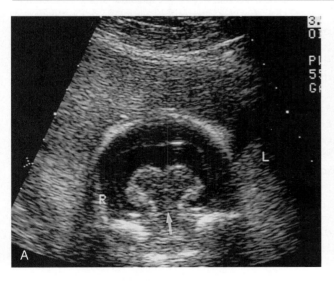

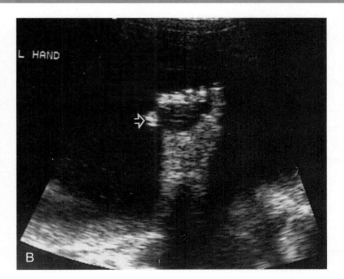

1. What is the most likely chromosomal anomaly associated with this second-trimester fetus (Figs. A and B)? Figure A is a coronal image of the fetal head. Figure B is an image of the left hand.

2. What percentage of fetuses with this chromosomal anomaly have cardiac abnormalities?

3. What extremity malformations are associated?

4. Name three associated facial malformations.

Pelvic Inflammatory Disease (Hydrosalpinx)

1. Figure A: bilateral adnexal masses (asterisks), fluid in the cul-de-sac (arrowheads). Figure B: tubular left adnexal structure. The most likely diagnosis is PID with left hydrosalpinx.

2. Transvaginal study.

3. No.

4. Yes. Partially treated but abnormal fallopian tubes are a high risk factor for a tubal pregnancy.

Reference

Soper DE: Upper genital tract infection. In Copeland LJ (ed): *Textbook of Gynecology.* Philadelphia, WB Saunders, 1993, pp 517–559.

Cross-Reference

Ultrasound: THE REQUISITES, pp 405–407.

Comment

The incidence of PID has increased in rate and in the number of hospitalizations. PID has also increased the rates of ectopic pregnancy and infertility. The economic consequences of PID are vast. More than 1 million women are treated for this disease in the United States each year, and more than 25% of these women are hospitalized annually with this diagnosis. As many as 150,000 women undergo surgical procedures for PID, some of which involve hysterectomies.

Typically, PID is clinically treated with antibiotics, and often an imaging study is not necessary. However, if the symptoms outlast or are worse than expected, an ultrasound examination is usually the first study to evaluate for the possibility of an abscess.

This case shows severe chronic PID (see Figs. A and B). Figure A shows complex bilateral adnexal masses (asterisks) and cul-de-sac fluid (arrows) posterior to the left adnexa. Figure B shows a typically dilated fallopian tube. When one tube in involved, it is almost always the same case with the other, even if not appreciated by imaging studies. Only in unusual cases of instrumentation or an intrauterine device is only one tube affected.

Although most cystic adnexal masses are ovarian in origin, an oval shape or an unusually complex mass should have several additional differential diagnoses, including infection, abscesses, and hydrosalpinges. If the hydrosalpinx contains internal echoes, it is probably infected (a pyosalpinx). On transabdominal study, it is not uncommon to only see an unusually oval-shaped mass. A transvaginal study is usually more definitive for detecting the true tubular nature of the mass. However, in this case, the transabdominal study made the correct diagnosis (see Fig. B).

Notes

Trisomy 13

1. Trisomy 13.

2. 50%.

3. Polydactyly and clubfoot.

4. Cleft lip/palate, cyclopia, and hypotelorism are among the facial malformations.

References

Hill LM: The sonographic detection of trisomies 13, 18, and 21. *Clin Obstet Gynecol* 39:831–850, 1996.

Lehman CD, Nyberg DA, Winter TC, et al: Trisomy 13 syndrome: Prenatal US findings in a review of 33 cases. *Radiology* 194:217–222, 1995.

Cross-Reference

Ultrasound: THE REQUISITES, p 217.

Comment

Trisomy 13 (Patau's syndrome) is a fatal chromosomal abnormality with many severe malformations associated. Compared with other trisomies, a high intrauterine spontaneous abortion rate accounts for its lower prevalence at birth. One large series reported that symmetric intrauterine growth restriction was present in almost half the cases; abnormal amniotic fluid was detected in almost one third, both oligohydramnios and polyhydramnios.

Neurologic malformations include holoprosencephaly (see Fig. A), microcephaly, enlarged cisterna magna, and hydrocephalus. Figure A shows a monoventrical with fused thalami (arrow) consistent with the most severe alobar form. Cleft lip/palate, cyclopia, and hypotelorism are among the facial malformations. Nuchal thickening, cystic hygroma, lymphangiectasia, and hydrops may be present.

The kidneys may be enlarged and are often hyperechoic (echogenic), with or without hydronephrosis. Omphalocele, bladder exstrophy, and echogenic (hyperechoic) bowel are additional abdominal abnormalities. Polydactyly (see Fig. B, open arrow = sixth digit), rocker-bottom or clubbed feet, and clenched/overlapping digits have been reported.

Cardiac defects can be seen in almost 50%. Hypoplastic left heart is common as well as ventriculoseptal defect. Single umbilical artery and papillary muscle calcification have also been reported in trisomy 13.

Notes

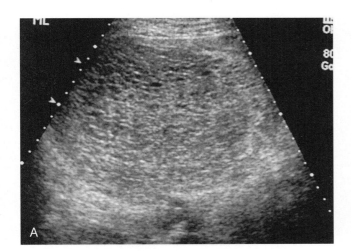

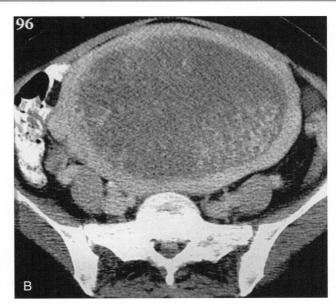

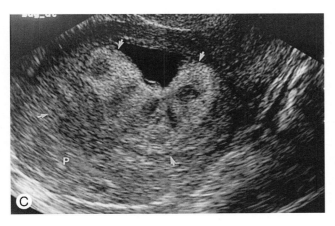

1. What is the pathologic spectrum of disease associated with the entity in this patient with a positive serum β-human chorionic gonadotropin (Figs. A and B). (Fig. A is an axial ultrasound [US] image of the uterus; Fig. B is the comparable image on a computed tomography [CT] scan.)

2. What is the classic US appearance?

3. What is the differential diagnosis of this second patient with a positive serum β-human chorionic gonadotropin (β-HCG) (Fig. C; P = placenta; arrows = heterogeneous area)?

4. What risk does a partial mole carry?

Gestational Trophoblastic Disease

1. Complete (see Figs. A and B) and partial (see Fig. C) hydatidiform mole, invasive mole, and chorio-carcinoma.

2. "Snowstorm" of tiny vesicles with increased through transmission expanding the endometrial canal.

3. Partial mole versus hydropic change of the placenta.

4. Chromosomal anomalies.

References

Carter J, Fowler J, Carlson J, et al: Transvaginal color flow Doppler sonography in the assessment of gestational trophoblastic disease. *J Ultrasound Med* 12:595–599, 1993.

Green CL, Angtuaco TL, Shah HR, et al: Gestational trophoblastic disease: A spectrum of radiologic diagnosis. *Radiographics* 16:1371–1384, 1996.

Cross-Reference

Ultrasound: THE REQUISITES, pp 333–335.

Comment

Several pathologic entities comprise the spectrum of gestational trophoblastic disease: a complete or partial hydatidiform mole, which comprises more than 80% of cases; an invasive mole; or choriocarcinoma (1% to 2% of cases). The first case (see Figs. A and B) shows the US and CT appearance of a complete hydatidiform mole.

The US appearance of gestational trophoblastic neoplasm has been described as an enlarged uterus with an irregular shape in some cases. The endometrium is expanded with a snowstorm appearance, which is caused by tiny vesicles that have increased through transmission (see Fig. A). If the vesicles enlarge, the appearance becomes more heterogeneous. US documentation of extension into the myometrium is important; myometrial nodules reflect invasion. Transvaginal scanning is helpful in assessing myometrial extension, and a demonstration of abnormal endometrial or myometrial flow with color or power Doppler can help to detect the tumor invasion. Magnetic resonance imaging also may be helpful in assessing uterine invasion of gestational trophoblastic neoplasia.

The second case (see Fig. C) is an example of a partial mole. A partial mole (arrows) forms within the placenta (P) of a coexistent fetus. The fetus is usually abnormal and has a high incidence of chromosomal anomalies. The differential diagnosis of this US appearance includes hydropic degeneration of the placenta. Once this finding is detected, a careful US analysis and karyotype of the fetus should be performed because multiple abnormalities and triploidy are common. Unlike a complete mole, the partial mole does not have malignant potential.

Notes

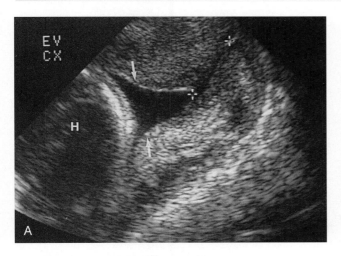

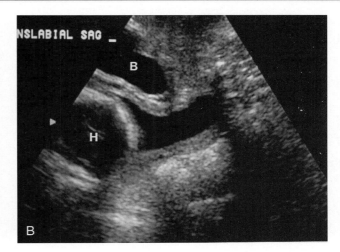

1. What is the diagnosis in these two third-trimester studies of the lower uterine segment (Figs. A and B; H = fetal head)? Figure A is a sagittal transvaginal image (+'s = closed endocervical length of 2.2 cm). Figure B is a sagittal translabial image (B = urinary bladder). Is either more severe and why?

2. Who is at increased risk for developing this problem?

3. What is the best technique for measuring the cervical length?

4. Which maneuver is most reliable to dilate a closed but incompetent cervix: coughing, standing, or transfundal pressure?

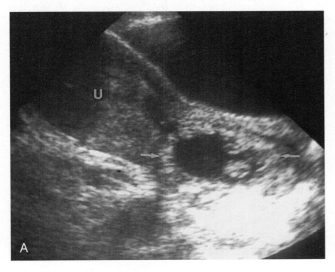

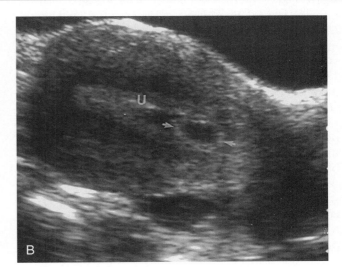

1. What are the most likely diagnoses of these gestational sacs (arrows) in these two cases (Figs. A and B; U = transabdominal sagittal images of the uterus)?

2. Why is the distinction so essential?

3. How is cervical ectopic pregnancy treated?

4. What accounts for the rising incidence of cervical ectopic pregnancies?

Incompetent Cervix

1. Figures A and B show an incompetent cervix. Figure B is worse, because it shows complete incompetence with bulging membranes.

2. Women who have a history of preterm labor or preterm delivery.

3. Transvaginal imaging.

4. Transfundal pressure.

Reference

Guzman ER, Pisatowski DM, Vintzileos AM, et al: A comparison of ultrasonographically detected cervical changes in response to transfundal pressure, coughing and standing in predicting cervical incompetence. *Am J Obstet Gynecol* 177:660–665, 1997.

Cross-Reference

Ultrasound: THE REQUISITES, pp 329–333.

Comment

Imaging of the lower uterine segment is an essential part of the obstetric ultrasound examination. The cervical length correlates inversely with the risk of preterm delivery (i.e., the longer the length, the less incidence of preterm delivery). Women with a prior history of preterm labor or delivery have an increased risk of premature labor in subsequent pregnancies.

The lower uterine segment can be imaged using a transabdominal, translabial, or transvaginal technique. Distention of the urinary bladder compresses the lower uterine segment to create the false appearance of a long cervix and the false appearance of a funneled cervix. Consequently, translabial and transvaginal imaging are more accurate when performed with a completely or almost completely empty urinary bladder.

Studies have shown that women with cervical incompetence demonstrate progressive cervical shortening on ultrasound over several weeks. In addition, application of transfundal pressure may dilate a closed cervix if the cervix is incompetent. This is a predictor that the cervix will progressively shorten through the gestation. Isolated opening of the internal os may not be detected by speculum or digital examination; ultrasound must be performed during transfundal pressure. The authors who studied transfundal pressure as a provocative maneuver use a 10 mm cervical length as the cutoff requiring cervical cerclage.

In these two cases, Figure A shows a cervix shortened to 2.2 cm, funneling of the internal os (arrows), with a V-shape to the funneling. Figure B shows only fluid distal the fetal head (H) without any demonstrable normal cervical tissue. On pelvic examination, this appears as bulging amniotic membranes seen in the vagina and loss of the pregnancy is almost always inevitable.

Notes

Cervical Ectopic Pregnancy

1. Figure A shows cervical implantation of the gestational sac (cervical ectopic pregnancy); Figure B shows an abortion in progress.

2. Treatment of a cervical ectopic pregnancy with dilatation and curettage can result in life-threatening hemorrhage.

3. Methotrexate, dilatation and evacuation following uterine artery ligation, or ultrasound-guided potassium chloride injection.

4. In vitro fertilization.

References

Frates MC, Benson CB, Doubilet PM, et al: Cervical ectopic pregnancy: Results of conservative treatment. *Radiology* 191:773–775, 1994.

Rosenberg RD, Williamson MR: Cervical ectopic pregnancy: Avoiding pitfalls in the ultrasound diagnosis. *J Ultrasound Med* 11:365–367, 1992.

Cross-Reference

Ultrasound: THE REQUISITES, p 418.

Comment

Cervical implantation of an ectopic pregnancy is among the rarest of sites, although, increasing in frequency with in vitro fertilization. Distinguishing this diagnosis from an abortion in progress is essential because simple dilatation and evacuation of a cervical ectopic pregnancy usually result in hemorrhage requiring a hysterectomy.

Patients with a cervical pregnancy usually present with bleeding, in one series between 5 and 8 weeks of gestational age. Ultrasound often demonstrates a normally shaped gestational sac in the lower uterine segment (as shown in Figure A), frequently with yolk sac and fetal heart activity. In an abortion in progress, the sac is malpositioned (as demonstrated by Figure B), usually abnormally shaped without any recognizable fetal pole or fetal heart motion. On a follow-up scan in 24 hours, an abortion in progress should show some change, but a cervical ectopic pregnancy will not.

In cases where there is no gestational sac, a heterogeneous mass may be seen in the lower uterine segment with a cervical implantation. In such cases, the differential diagnosis includes entities such as pedunculated degenerating myoma, abortion in progress, or vascularized retained products of conception (RPOC). Detection of high diastolic flow, proposed as an indicator of cervical ectopic pregnancy can also be seen with RPOC and gestational trophoblastic disease.

Notes

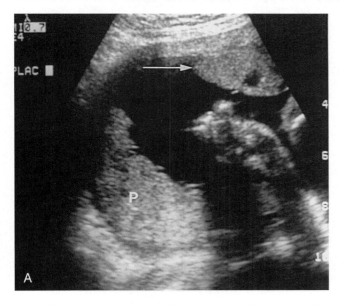

1. What is the abnormality (arrow) shown in this image of the uterus in a late second-trimester pregnancy (Fig. A)? P = Placenta.

2. What is the etiology?

3. What is a possible perinatal complication?

4. What is a potential postnatal complication?

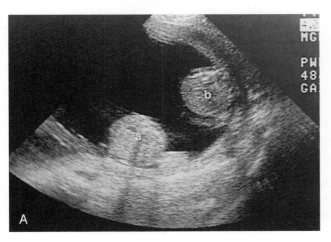

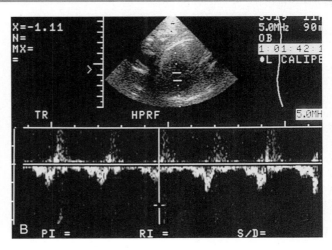

1. In this late second-trimester twin pregnancy, fetus "a" is freely moving, and fetus "b" remains in a fixed position (Fig. A). What is the most likely diagnosis?

2. What is the term used to describe the twin in this syndrome affected by oligohydramnios, and what is the likely prognosis?

3. What are the ultrasound criteria used to define this syndrome?

4. In another twin pregnancy with the same syndrome, in the late third trimester, what is detected in the freely moving twin on this spectral Doppler evaluation of its right atrium (Fig. B)?

Succenturiate Lobe

1. Succenturiate lobe of the placenta.

2. Failure of normal villous atrophy.

3. Hemorrhage.

4. Retained placenta with hemorrhage or infection.

References

Hata K, Hata T, Aoki S, et al: Succenturiate placenta diagnosed by ultrasound. *Gynecol Obstet Invest* 25:273–276, 1988.

Nelson LH, Fishburne JI, Stearns BR: Ultrasonographic description of a succenturiate placenta. *Obstet Gynecol* 49(Suppl):79–80, 1977.

Cross-Reference

Ultrasound: THE REQUISITES, p 313.

Comment

This case demonstrates a rare but important placental abnormality—the presence of a succenturiate lobe. This is defined as an accessory placental lobe that is removed from but in vascular continuity with the main placenta. Fetal vessels under the amniochorionic membranes connect this accessory lobe to the main placenta. This anomaly is reported to occur in up to 0.28% of pregnancies. The etiology is a regional failure of placental villi to atrophy.

Despite its rarity, this is a very important abnormality to detect on prenatal ultrasound. Sonography can detect and localize the accessory placenta. If not detected, several serious complications can ensue. Prenatally and during labor, the connecting vessels can rupture, leading to life-threatening fetal hemorrhage. A vaso previa (fetal hemorrhage) can develop at time of labor and delivery if these vessels are over the internal cervical os. If the succenturiate lobe is not delivered, it can lead to postpartum maternal hemorrhage and infection. A succenturiate lobe should be suspected at the time of delivery if severed fetal vessels are present at the torn edge of the membranes of the placenta.

Notes

Twin-Twin Transfusion

1. Twin-twin transfusion syndrome.

2. Adherence of the "donor" twin in its sac, called the "stuck twin syndrome." The prognosis is poor.

3. Monochorionic placenta, same gender, marked growth discordance (>20%), polyhydramnios in the larger twin sac and oligohydramnios in the smaller twin sac.

4. Tricuspid regurgitation.

Acknowledgment

Figure A for Case 93 courtesy of Beryl Benacerraf, MD.

Reference

Bruner JP, Rosemond RL: Twin-twin transfusion syndrome: A subset of the twin oligohydramnios-polyhydramnios sequence. *Am J Obstet Gynecol* 169:925–930, 1993.

Cross-Reference

Ultrasound: THE REQUISITES, pp 349–351.

Comment

The twin-twin transfusion (TTT) syndrome is a serious complication of monochorionic gestations. It is strictly defined by interconnecting placental vessels between the two twins, which result in umbilical arteriovenous shunting of blood from one twin to the other. When significant shunting occurs, one twin (donor) becomes small with anemia and oligohydramnios. The other twin (recipient) enlarges and develops polycythemia, volume overload, and heart failure, as well as polyhydramnios. In its most severe form, the smaller twin can become stuck to the intervening membrane, with very high mortality (see Fig. A).

Ultrasound criteria for the TTT include a monochorionic twinning (a monochorionic [fused] placenta), twins of the same gender, and a growth discordance between the twins of at least 20%. Polyhydramnios is often present in the larger sac with oligohydramnios present in the smaller sac. Oligohydramnios may be so severe that the "stuck" fetus may be very difficult to identify.

The recipient twin is subject to several complications. Cardiomegaly results from biventricular hypertrophy and dilatation. Tricuspid regurgitation is often present (see Fig. B). If the donor twin dies, the recipient can suffer an embolic phenomenon through the arteriovenous connections, resulting in cerebral damage. Color Doppler evaluation of the placenta has largely failed to identify the significant vascular connections.

Notes

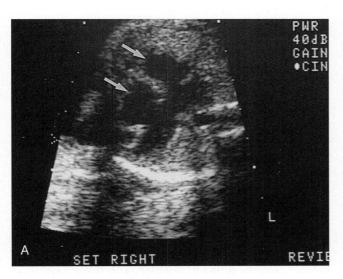

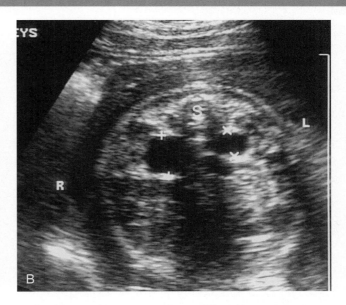

1. What is the finding in this axial image of the heart in this second-trimester fetus (Fig. A; arrows = ventricles)? What is the most likely chromosomal anomaly?

2. What is the abnormality noted in this axial image of the fetal abdomen in the same fetus (Fig. B; + = renal pelves; R = right; L = left)? Is your suspicion for the karyotype abnormality thought to be present increased?

3. What cardiac finding has recently been seen with higher frequency in this disorder?

4. What pelvic abnormality on prenatal ultrasound has been described in Down syndrome?

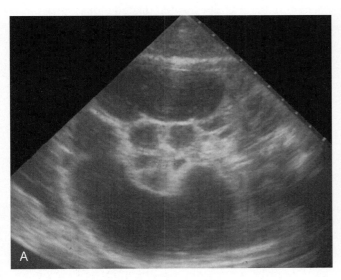

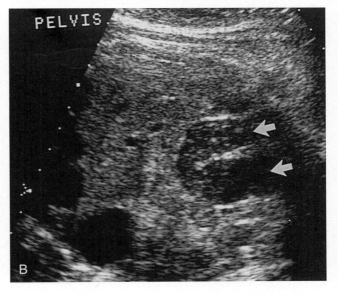

1. In these two third-trimester fetuses, which portion of the bowel is dilated (Fig. A, a midabdominal axial image; Fig. B, a coronal image of the fetal body; arrows = one of the bowel loops)?

2. What is the most common cause of colon obstruction in the *neonate*?

3. Is oligohydramnios or polyhydramnios usually present on prenatal ultrasound with Hirschsprung's disease?

4. What is the amniotic fluid status with anorectal atresia?

C A S E   9 4

Trisomy 21 (Down Syndrome)—Advanced

1. Atrioventricular (AV) canal. Trisomy 21.

2. Pelviectasis. Yes.

3. Intraventricular echogenic focus.

4. Widening of the iliac angle.

References

Kliewer MA, Hertzberg BS, Freed KS, et al: Dysmorphologic features of the fetal pelvis in Down syndrome: Prenatal sonographic depiction and diagnostic importance of the iliac angle. *Radiology* 201:681–684, 1996.

Winter TC, Reichman JA, Luna JA, et al: Frontal lobe shortening in second-trimester fetuses with trisomy 21: Usefulness as a US marker. *Radiology* 207:215–222, 1998.

Cross-Reference

Ultrasound: THE REQUISITES, pp 221, 275.

Comment

Various ultrasound findings have been described in trisomy 21. A short humerus and femur, dilatation of the renal pelves (see Fig. B), and hyperechoic (echogenic) bowel can be seen. Three new markers have been reported in the radiology literature. An echogenic focus in the ventricle of the heart, papillary muscle calcification, is seen more frequently in fetuses with Down syndrome. This calcification is present histologically in 15% to 17% of aneuploid fetuses versus 2% to 5% of normals. The significance of this finding is controversial, particularly if it is the only abnormality on a prenatal ultrasound. In a *high-risk* population, a statistically significant association has been shown with Down syndrome.

Widening of the iliac angle in the pelvis correlates with the pelvic flaring that is characteristic of this syndrome. The iliac wing angle is measured on a transverse view of the pelvis, using the angle formed by the two iliac crests. The iliac angle is measured between 15 and 20 weeks, and the mean measurement is 75 degrees in Down syndrome versus 60 degrees in normal fetuses. However, the iliac angle varies with the level at which it is measured, and there is a large overlap between normal fetuses and those with Down syndrome.

The frontal lobe of the brain has been shown to be shorter in Down syndrome compared with normal fetuses. The frontothalamic distance can be measured on prenatal ultrasound in the second trimester, from the calvarial table of the frontal lobe to the posterior margin of the thalamus.

Notes

C A S E   9 5

Hirschsprung's Disease

1. Colon.

2. Hirschsprung's disease.

3. Polyhydramnios.

4. Usually normal or decreased.

Reference

Vermesh M, Mayden KL, Confino E, et al: Prenatal sonographic diagnosis of Hirschsprung's disease *J Ultrasound Med* 5:37–39, 1986.

Cross-Reference

Ultrasound: THE REQUISITES, pp 258–262.

Comment

Hirschsprung's disease is the most common cause of colon obstruction in the neonate. The differential diagnosis of neonatal colon obstruction includes meconium plug syndrome (small left colon) and anal atresia. Hirschsprung's disease is caused by failed caudal migration of ganglion cells to the rectosigmoid wall. Ganglion cells are absent from both Auerbach's and Meissner's plexuses, leading to continuous contraction of the muscle. Chromosomal anomalies are infrequently associated, most commonly with Down syndrome.

When prenatal ultrasound demonstrates dilated bowel, it is important to distinguish dilated colon from dilated small bowel. This can sometimes be difficult. However, there are helpful signs to diagnose large bowel dilatation. Peripherally located dilated loops, particularly the ascending and descending colon (Fig. A), are common. A U- or V- shaped loop of bowel can be detected, particularly in rectosigmoid distention (see Fig. B, arrows). Peristalsis is commonly lacking. Other nonspecific findings include increased abdominal distention, and polyhydramnios has been reported with Hirschsprung's disease on prenatal ultrasound. In anorectal atresia, however, the amniotic fluid volume is either normal or decreased.

When colon obstruction is suspected, the primary concern is for anorectal atresia with its frequent additional anomalies. However, Hirschsprung's disease is also a possibility. It has no associated anomalies.

When Hirschsprung's disease is suspected, a barium enema should be performed in the neonatal period. Neonates with Hirschsprung's disease usually present after 24 hours with vomiting, abdominal distention and failure to pass meconium. Complications include bowel perforation and necrotizing enterocolitis, which can lead to sepsis. The diagnosis is made by a full-thickness rectal biopsy.

Notes

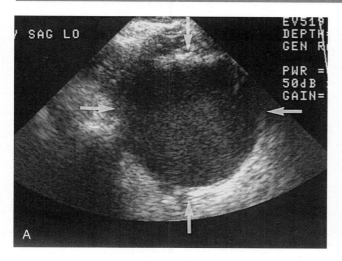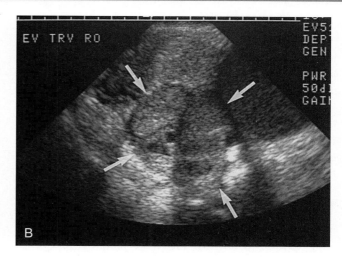

1. In this 31-year-old woman with bilateral pelvic "fullness" on bimanual pelvic examination, what are the ultrasound findings and the most likely diagnosis in this case (Figs. A and B; arrows identify the ovaries)?

2. Is there a characteristic appearance of an endometrioma on an ultrasound examination? If not, what is the most common appearance?

3. Is ultrasound sensitive in the detection of abnormalities in this entity?

4. Does endometriosis adversely affect fertility?

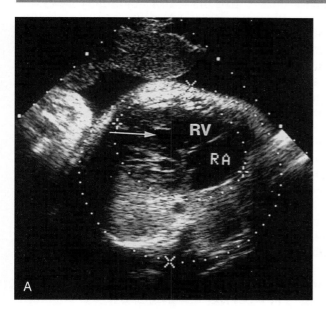

1. In this axial view of the fetal chest, the four-chamber view of the heart is shown (Fig. A). What is the most likely cause of the ventricular discordance? RA = right atrium; RV = right ventricle; arrow = left ventricle.

2. Which ventricle is enlarged with coarctation of the aorta?

3. Which ventricle is enlarged with a ductus occlusion?

4. Which ventricle is enlarged with intrauterine growth restriction?

Endometriosis

1. Bilateral complex ovarian masses. Bilateral hemorrhagic lesions, most likely endometriomas.

2. No. Homogeneous, low level echoes.

3. No; ultrasound identifies only 11%.

4. Yes.

References

Friedman H, Vogelzang RL, Mendelson EB, et al: Endometriosis detection by US with laparoscopic correlation. *Radiology* 157:217–220, 1985.

Kupfer MC, Schwimer SR, Lebovic J: Transvaginal sonographic appearance of endometriomata: Spectrum of findings. *J Ultrasound Med* 11:129–133, 1992.

Outwater E, Schiebler ML, Owen RS, et al: Characterization of hemorrhagic adnexal lesions with MR imaging: Blinded reader study. *Radiology* 186:489–494, 1993.

Cross-Reference

Ultrasound: THE REQUISITES, p 403.

Comment

Endometriosis is a disorder in which benign endometrial glands and stroma are located outside of the uterus. The diagnosis is made definitively with laparoscopy. Implants of endometrial tissue are commonly seen on the ovary, uterus, and ligament in the cul-de-sac and can be found on the rectosigmoid colon. If small, these implants are not seen with ultrasound, accounting for the low sensitivity of ultrasound to detect endometriosis. Magnetic resonance imaging (MRI) has been shown to be more sensitive because of the ability to detect small endometriomas (<1 cm) and to accurately characterize blood based on signal intensity. In addition, MRI can reveal implants or evidence of hemosiderin along the peritoneum and adhesions that are the sequela of endometriosis.

The endometrioma is a cyst that contains altered blood, which usually arises from an ovary and is often bilateral, as shown here. On ultrasound, endometriomas usually have internal echoes and often demonstrate homogeneous low-level echoes (see Fig. A). The internal material can be hyperechoic (see Fig. B). Internal septations or fluid-fluid levels may be present.

Using MRI, endometriomas are often hyperintense on T_1-weighted images. On T_2-weighted sequences, they may demonstrate a relative decrease in signal intensity ("shading") or they can be hyperintense. The presence of shading is the most accurate criterion to distinguish an endometrioma from other hemorrhagic or nonhemorrhagic adnexal masses.

Notes

Ventricular Discordance

1. Hypoplastic left heart.

2. Right.

3. Right.

4. Right.

References

Brown DL, DiSalvo DN, Frates MC, et al: Sonography of the fetal heart: Normal variants and pitfalls. *AJR Am J Roentgenol* 160:1251–1255, 1993.

Weil SR, Huhta JC: Sonographic differential diagnosis of fetal cardiac abnormalities. *Semin Ultrasound CT MR* 14:298–317, 1993.

Cross-Reference

Ultrasound: THE REQUISITES, pp 240–243.

Comment

The four-chamber heart view is standard in any obstetric ultrasound screening examination. Although anomalies can be missed using this view only, the sizes of the ventricles are very important and can indicate various cardiac malformations. An important normal variant is a prominent moderator band. This hypoechoic to isoechoic (relative to myocardium) band of tissue in the apex of the right ventricle makes the ventricular cavity appear smaller than the left in the normal heart. The apices of both ventricles should normally extend to the cardiac apex in a true four-chamber view. The ventricles typically measure 1:1, and the measurement is obtained just behind the atrioventricular valves.

In the normal fetus, the right ventricular width mildly increases compared with the left with advancing gestational age, which is an important anatomic relationship to recognize. However, enlargement or diminution of the left ventricle can indicate various cardiac malformations. If the left ventricle is small with the right ventricle enlarged, left-sided obstructing lesions should be considered. Coarctation of the aorta or the more severe hypoplastic left heart (shown in this case) and interrupted aortic arch cause diminution of the left ventricle. Additional causes of small left ventricle with right ventricular enlargement include a double-outlet right ventricle.

A small left ventricle has also been reported with intrauterine growth restriction in fetuses that also develop right ventricular dilatation; this results from redistribution of blood flow to the fetal head with increased venous return to the right side of the heart.

Enlargement of the left ventricle with a normal right ventricle usually indicates left ventricular myocardial dysfunction. Specifically, critical aortic stenosis and primary endocardial fibroelastosis should be considered.

Notes

Challenge

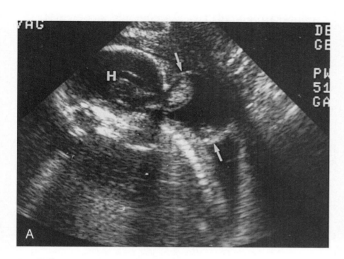

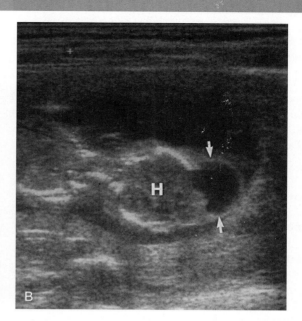

1. What entity is shown by arrows in these two second-trimester fetuses (Fig. A, sagittal fetal head and neck; Fig. B, coronal fetal head)?

2. Would the α-fetoprotein (AFP) level usually be elevated in these cases?

3. What is Meckel-Gruber syndrome?

4. What is the prognosis in this case?

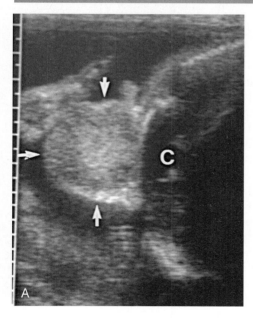

1. In a third-trimester fetus, what is the differential diagnosis of this facial abnormality (arrows) arising from the check (c) on this oblique image (Fig. A)? Which diagnosis is favored considering its echogenicity and compressibility by fetal limbs on real-time observation?

2. Which tumor may arise in the brain and extend into the face?

3. What is the significance of associated polyhydramnios?

4. What is the differential diagnosis of a mass arising from the inside of the mouth?

Encephalocele

1. Encephalocele.

2. No.

3. Microcephaly with an occipital meningoencephalocele, enlarged kidneys with cystic renal dysplasia, hepatic fibrosis, and polydactyly.

4. Poor.

Reference
Goldstein RB, LaPidus AS, Filly RA: Fetal cephaloceles: Diagnosis with US. *Radiology* 180:803–808, 1991.

Cross-Reference
Ultrasound: THE REQUISITES, pp 218–219.

Comment
Encephaloceles are midline cranial defects that occur in approximately 1 in 10,000 pregnancies. A cephalocele describes a herniation of central nervous system (CNS) meninges through the midline defect in the cranium. They may contain only cerebrospinal fluid (CSF) (cranial meningocele) or brain and CSF fluid (encephalocele). Both have a poor prognosis. For an encephalocele, the mortality rate is estimated at 50%, and 75% of the survivors are mentally retarded. Both types have associated anomalies: CNS (up to 75%), systemic (70%), and karyotype (44%).

All encephaloceles, except those secondary to amniotic band syndrome, are midline. In the Western World, most encephaloceles (80%) occur in the occipital region (see Fig. A); frontal and parietal (see Fig. B) locations comprise the remaining 20%. Frontal cephaloceles, more common in the Eastern World, have a better prognosis.

The ultrasound appearance of an encephalocele may be entirely cystic (see Fig. B), cystic and solid (see Fig. A), cyst-within-a-cyst, or predominantly solid. The cranial defect is present but is not always apparent. Secondary findings include microcephaly, lemon-head deformity (30%), beaked tectum (70%), and ventriculomegaly (50%). Associated CNS anomalies include migrational abnormalities, agenesis of the corpus callosum, and cerebellar abnormalities.

Associated non-neurologic malformations include intrauterine growth restriction and abnormalities of amniotic fluid volume. Cardiac anomalies, facial clefts, and renal cystic disease have been reported.

Unlike myelomeningoceles, the AFP level is usually not elevated with encephalocele, because skin covers the anomaly.

Notes

Facial Mass

1. Hemangioma, lymphangioma, teratoma, neurofibroma, granular cell tumor (epulis), retinoblastoma, dacryocystocele, mucocele, cyst, and malignant melanoma. The most likely diagnosis is hemangioma.

2. Teratoma.

3. Worsened outcome.

4. Gingival granular cell tumor (oropharyngeal epulis), teratoma, or simple cyst.

Reference
Shipp TD, Bromley B, Benacerraf B: The ultrasound appearance and outcome for fetuses with masses distorting the fetal face. *J Ultrasound Med* 14:673–678, 1995.

Cross-Reference
Ultrasound: THE REQUISITES, pp 215–218.

Comment
Facial masses are rare fetal anomalies. They can arise from any region of the face (e.g., nose, orbit, oropharynx) or from the neck or brain and extend to involve the face. The differential diagnosis includes benign (e.g., hemangioma, lymphangioma, gingival granular cell tumor [epulis], teratoma, neurofibroma, dacryocystocele, mucocele, cyst) and malignant lesions (e.g., teratoma, retinoblastoma, melanoma).

The location may aid in determining the etiology. With large masses, it can be difficult to accurately determine its site of origin. Hemangiomas usually arise from the scalp or skin. They are often soft, easily compressible, and often of uniform echogenicity (see Fig. A).

Masses that arise from the mouth include the gingival granular cell tumor (congenital epulis), teratoma, or simple cyst. The teratoma is the most common mass in neonates. It can arise from many regions of the head and neck (e.g., nose, palate, thyroid, neck, brain). A dacryocystocele is a dilatation of the lacrimal duct. Retinoblastoma arises from the globe.

Color Doppler may be useful in tumors that may have high flow (e.g. teratomas) and also in malignancies.

The outcomes depend on the histopathology of the mass and the extent of head and neck involvement. Hemangiomas and granular cell tumors may be completely excised. Teratomas that arise in the brain and extend into the face have a uniformly poor prognosis; they generally destroy the intracranial structures. A dacryocystocele can resolve without treatment.

Detection of polyhydramnios in association with one of the masses carries a poor prognosis, because it often suggests an obstruction to swallowing.

Notes

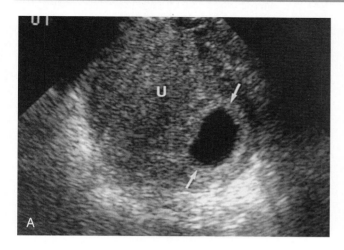

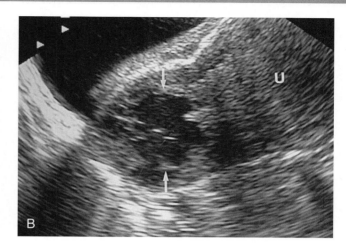

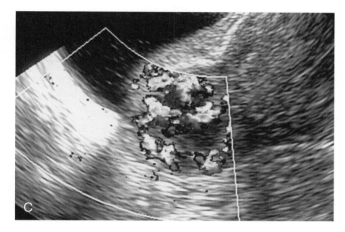

1. Two cases with the same early first-trimester diagnosis. U = uterus; arrows = gestational sacs. Figure A shows the transvaginal image of patient A; Figure B shows the transabdominal image of patient B. Figure C is the color Doppler evaluation of Figure B. What is the diagnosis?

2. What entities can cause a gestational sac to appear eccentric?

3. What is the interstitial line sign?

4. What is Ruge-Simon syndrome?

Cornual (Interstitial) Ectopic Pregnancy

1. Cornual ectopic pregnancies.

2. Cornual ectopic, myoma, myometrial contraction, bicornuate uterus, and septate uterus.

3. A thin hyperechoic line extending from the central endometrial stripe to the periphery of the ectopic cornual gestational sac.

4. A cornual ectopic that rotates the uterus, making the sac appear to be centrally located.

References

Ackerman TE, Levi CS, Dashefsky SM, et al: Interstitial line: Sonographic finding in interstitial (cornual) ectopic pregnancy. *Radiology* 189:83–87, 1993.

Frates MC, Laing FC: Sonographic evaluation of ectopic pregnancy: An update. *AJR Am J Roentgenol* 165:251–259, 1995.

Cross-Reference

Ultrasound: THE REQUISITES, pp 418, 420.

Comment

An interstitial or cornual ectopic pregnancy is an unusual form of ectopic implantation. Because of the proximity of the interstitial portion of the tube to the uterine cavity, the diagnosis can be challenging. Patients present later than the typical ectopic pregnancy, as late as the beginning of the second trimester. The cornua is partially protected by the myometrium and is capable of expanding more than the remainder of the tube to accommodate an enlarging gestational sac. As a result of late presentation, a rupture can be catastrophic and can lead occasionally to life-threatening hemorrhage.

The ectopic gestational sac is usually eccentrically located (see Figs. A and B) in a cornual ectopic. Ruge-Simon syndrome refers to the rare occurrence of a cornual ectopic pregnancy that does not appear eccentric because the uterus has rotated. Uterine anomalies such as septate or bicornuate uterus can also result in an eccentric sac location. Focal myometrial contractions, leiomyomata, and a retroverted uterus result in a similar appearance. Although some literature suggests that a myometrium less than 5 mm surrounding the sac indicates a cornual ectopic, this was found to be an unreliable indicator in one important study. The absence of surrounding myometrium would suggest an interstitial pregnancy; however, the apparent presence of myometrium around the sac does not exclude it. This is shown in a cornual ectopic pregnancy in a third patient in a transvaginal coronal image (Fig. D; +'s showing the apparent myometrium). The ectopic pregnancy may be a live fetus (see Fig. D) or a mass of solid, vascularized tissue (see Fig. C).

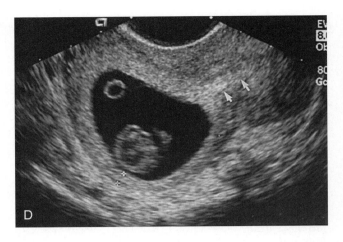

The interstitial line sign (see Fig. D; arrow = endometrium) has been reported as an important finding in a cornual ectopic pregnancy; a straight, thin hyperechoic line extends from the endometrium to the ectopically placed gestational sac. It is thought to represent either the interstitial portion of the fallopian tube or the endometrial canal. This sign has been shown to be more sensitive than either the eccentric sac location or myometrial thinning in confirming the presence of a cornual ectopic pregnancy.

Notes

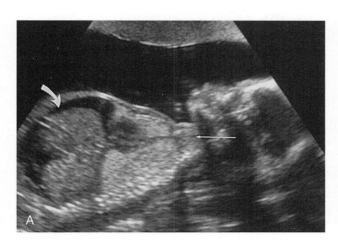

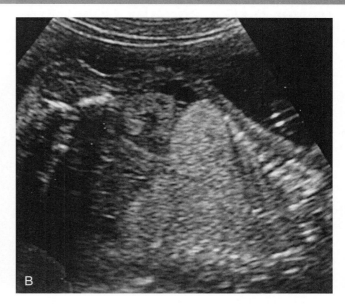

1. In this late second-trimester fetus, what is the differential diagnosis of bilateral lung abnormality shown in Figures A (sagittal) and B (coronal) of the fetal chest? In Figure A, what do the straight and curved arrows denote?

2. What causes the increased echogenicity of the lungs in laryngotracheal obstruction?

3. Are the lungs pathologically immature, developmentally normal, or of advanced maturity?

4. What is Fraser's syndrome?

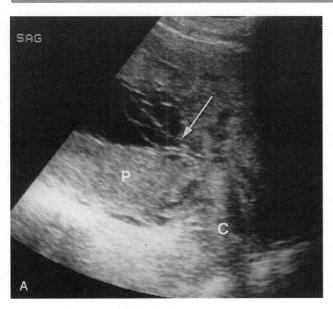

1. What is the problem, and what are risk factors for the abnormality shown on this prenatal sonogram of the lower uterine segment near term (Fig. A; arrow = cord insertion; P = placenta; C = cervix)?

2. What are the clinical indicators?

3. What fetal monitoring is conducted once this condition is diagnosed?

4. What is the treatment?

Laryngotracheal Obstruction

1. Laryngotracheal obstruction, bilateral cystic adenomatoid malformation type III, and sequestration (rare). Straight arrow = fluid-filled trachea; curved arrow = ascites.

2. Alveolar distention with fluid.

3. Advanced maturity.

4. Tracheal or bronchial stenosis, renal agenesis, microphthalmia, cryptophthalmos, and polydactyly or syndactyly.

References

De Hullu JA, Kornman LH, Beekhuis JR, Nikkels PGJ: The hyperechogenic lungs of laryngotracheal obstruction. *Ultrasound Obstet Gynecol* 6:372-272, 1995.

Kassanos D, Christodoulou CN, Agapitos E, et al: Prenatal ultrasonographic detection of the tracheal atresia sequence. *Ultrasound Obstet Gynecol* 10:133-136, 1997.

Cross-Reference

Ultrasound: THE REQUISITES, pp 247-248.

Comment

Fetal laryngotracheal obstruction is a severe, uncommon anomaly with a grave prognosis. Associated syndromes include Fraser's syndrome (described above), vertebral defects, imperforate anus, tracheoesophageal fistula, radial and renal dysplasia, and limb anomalies (VATER), DiGeorge developmental field defect, and rhizomelic chondrodysplasia punctata.

On prenatal ultrasound, the lungs appear uniformly enlarged and hyperechoic (see Figs. A and B). This is due to expansion of the alveoli with fluid. A secondary mass effect may be present, with compression of the diaphragm, heart, and mediastinal structures. Fetal ascites and polyhydramnios can develop, probably due to obstruction of the esophagus and venous return to the heart (see Fig. A). Oligohydramnios has been described in one case. In addition, a dilated, fluid-filled tracheobronchial tree below the level of obstruction has been described in at least one case and definitively proves the diagnosis if detected (see Fig. A).

Pathologically, the lungs show advanced maturity. The expansion of airspaces with fluid induces alveolar proliferation, which accounts for the advanced maturity.

Most fetuses die at birth owing to respiratory distress. Monitoring with ultrasound throughout the pregnancy has been advised, as well as delivery at a center where emergent tracheostomy or laryngotracheoplasty could be performed.

Notes

Obligate Cord

1. Obligate presentation of the umbilical cord. Breech positioning and small fetuses, particularly if premature.

2. Fetal heart decelerations during uterine contractions.

3. Nonstress tests and follow-up ultrasounds.

4. Surgery: cesarean section delivery.

References

Pelosi MA: Antepartum ultrasonic diagnosis of cord presentation. *Am J Obstet Gynecol* 162:599-601, 1990.

Sakamoto H, Takagi K, Masaoka N, et al: Clinical application of the perineal scan: Prepartum screening for cord presentation. *Am J Obstet Gynecol* 155:1041-1043, 1986.

Cross-Reference

Ultrasound: THE REQUISITES, p 313.

Comment

Obligate presentation of the cord refers to presentation of the umbilical cord before the fetus at the time of birth. The condition is more common in the setting of a breech positioning (particularly a footling breech) as well as small fetuses, including those delivered prematurely. Other risk factors include multiple gestations, polyhydramnios, multiparity, disproportion, incompetent cervix, and "hourglass membranes." Diagnosis of this condition is essential, because prolapse of the cord into the cervix during delivery can be catastrophic for the fetus. In addition, the positioning of the cord results in cord compression and variable fetal cardiac decelerations or bradycardia during uterine contractions.

Diagnosis can be made at the time of delivery by palpation; the umbilical cord can be palpated in the lower uterine segment on pelvic digital examination in some cases. An antenatal diagnosis has also been made with ultrasound. As this case demonstrates, the umbilical cord will be identified overlying the internal os (see Fig. A). Transperineal scanning is helpful to image the lower uterine segment and determine the presenting part.

If diagnosed prenatally, a management scheme has been outlined. Nonstress fetal cardiac monitoring is performed at weekly intervals or more frequently if clinically warranted. Application of fundal and suprapubic pressure may provoke fetal bradycardia, indicating cord entrapment. If the cord remains in a presenting position, prompt delivery by cesarean section is required at term.

Notes

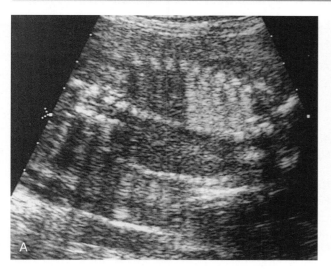

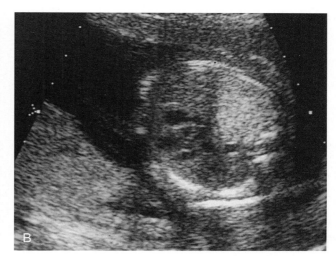

1. What is the differential diagnosis of the isolated left-sided hyperechoic (echogenic) abnormality shown in the chest of this mid–second-trimester fetus? Figure A is a coronal image, and Figure B is an axial image of the fetal chest.

2. What lesion may have systemic arterial supply?

3. Which type of congenital diaphragmatic hernia (CDH) appears as a solid mass?

4. What accounts for the echogenicity of the lung in bronchial obstruction or atresia?

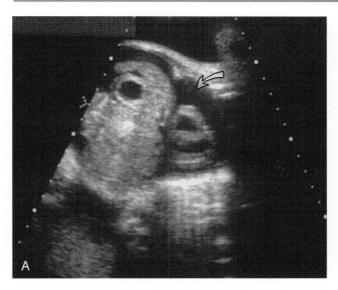

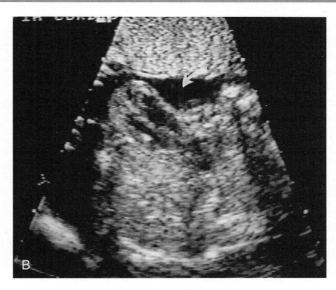

1. What rare anomaly is demonstrated in the axial images of the fetal chest in these two cases (Figs. A and B)? The curved arrows point to amniotic fluid.

2. What is the most common location?

3. Are chromosomal defects associated?

4. What are the most common intracardiac anomalies associated?

CASE 103

Mucous Plug

1. Sequestration, cystic adenomatoid malformation type III, or mucous plug/bronchial atresia.

2. Extralobar or intralobar sequestration.

3. Right-sided hernias containing liver.

4. Alveolar distention with fluid.

Reference

Meizner I, Rosenak D: The vanishing fetal intrathoracic mass: Consider an obstructing mucous plug. *Ultrasound Obstet Gynecol* 6:275–277, 1995.

Cross-Reference

Ultrasound: THE REQUISITES, pp 247–249.

Comment

A laryngotracheal obstruction presents on an antenatal ultrasound with enlarged, bilaterally hyperechoic lungs. The only differential consideration would be bilateral cystic adenomatoid malformation (CAM) type III or sequestrations. Bronchial atresia or an obstruction with a mucous plug can cause an isolated region of obstructed lung to enlarge and increase in echogenicity, which is demonstrated by this case. On prenatal ultrasound, a hyperechoic pulmonary mass is seen, raising the possibility of several diagnoses: CAM, sequestration, and CDH containing liver or other solid organ (if right-sided).

A focal hyperechoic lung "mass" due to bronchial obstruction is caused by distended alveoli that contain fluid. Pathologically, the lung tissue shows advanced maturity, with alveolar proliferation induced by fluid distention of the airspace. The enlarged region of lung may cause a mass effect and a mediastinal shift. Detection of branching bronchi within this region would assist in making an accurate diagnosis.

An improvement or a relative decrease in the size of a hyperechoic lung mass, and even resolution, have been described on prenatal ultrasound with several entities: CAM, sequestration, and CDH (except for those with intestine or stomach). These have been reported to improve in case reports or small series. In addition, obstruction of a bronchus with a mucous plug can cause a hyperechoic mass that improves or resolves in utero.

Notes

CASE 104

Ectopia Cordis

1. Ectopia cordis (the heart outside the thorax).

2. Thoracic.

3. Yes.

4. Conotruncal anomalies.

Acknowledgment
Figure B for Case 104 courtesy of Dennis Wood.

References

Hornberger LK, Colan SD, Lock JE, et al: Outcome of patients with ectopia cordis and significant intracardiac defects. *Circulation* 94:32–37, 1996.

Liang RI, Huang SE, Chang FM: Prenatal diagnosis of ectopia cordis at 10 weeks of gestation using two-dimensional and three-dimensional ultrasonography. *Ultrasound Obstet Gynecol* 10(2):137–139, 1997.

Cross-Reference

Ultrasound: THE REQUISITES, pp 269–270.

Comment

Ectopia cordis is defined as partial or complete displacement of the heart outside the thorax. The heart is most commonly located adjacent to the thorax (60%). However, the heart can exist outside the body cavity in other locations: abdominal (30%), thoracoabdominal (7%), or even cervical (3%). Ectopia cordis is one of the malformations that constitute the pentalogy of Cantrell, which also includes congenital cardiac defects, a supraumbilical omphalocele, a distal sternal cleft, and ventral diaphragmatic hernia.

The ultrasound diagnosis can be made as early as the first trimester and is always made by the second trimester. The fetal heart is seen outside the thorax, as shown by these two cases. Because of the associated malformations in the pentalogy of Cantrell, a careful evaluation must be made for other anomalies. In addition to these midline malformations, cranial anomalies, cleft lip and palate, gastrointestinal and genitourinary abnormalities, and pulmonary hypoplasia have been associated.

The prognosis is serious for infants with ectopia cordis, particularly the thoracic type. The associated cardiac malformations, which are most commonly conotruncal anomalies, account for the poor outcome. One series of infants with ectopia cordis has been reported; two thirds of the infants survived beyond the newborn period following surgical correction of the cardiac defects, which included tetralogy of Fallot and a double-outlet right ventricle with a ventriculoseptal defect.

Notes

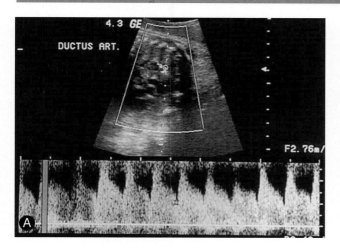
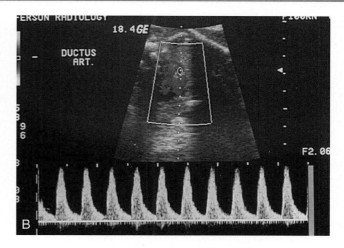

1. In this early third-trimester fetus, Figure A was taken one day before Figure B. What does a decreased ductal pulsatility index (see Fig. A) indicate? What has happened between the two studies?

2. Between which two structures and in which direction does the ductus arteriosus flow?

3. What medication used in pregnancy causes ductal constriction?

4. What ultrasound view shows the ductus arch as a "hockey-stick" configuration?

Ductus Arteriosus

1. Constriction of the ductus. Resolution of the constriction.

2. The pulmonary artery to the aorta.

3. Indomethacin.

4. Sagittal.

Reference

Sherer D, Divon M: Prenatal ultrasonographic assessment of the ductus arteriosus: A review. *Obstet Gynecol* 87:630–637, 1996.

Cross-Reference

Ultrasound: THE REQUISITES, pp 237–243.

Comment

The fetal ductus arteriosus connects the pulmonary trunk to the aorta. Oxygenated blood is delivered via umbilical veins through the umbilical portion of the left portal vein in the liver to the right side of the heart. The blood then flows from the right side of the heart via the pulmonary trunk and ductus arteriosus to the descending aorta. Additionally, oxygenated blood flows through the foramen ovale into the left atrium, left ventricle, and ascending aorta to supply the head and upper extremities.

An ultrasound evaluation of the ductus is important in women receiving indomethacin, a prostaglandin inhibitor, for tocolysis. Figure A shows abnormal ductus flow in a patient who took a large number of indomethacin tablets. Figure B demonstrates the resumption of a normal ductus waveform after the medication was stopped. Short-term use causes reversible mild constriction in ductal flow. However, long-term use can cause ductal constriction that results in significant secondary tricuspid regurgitation. Constriction of the ductus is detected by a decrease in the pulsatility index (<1.9), as shown in Figure A.

Using prenatal ultrasound, the ductus arteriosus is evaluated in sagittal and oblique/transverse views. The sagittal view shows the ductus as a hockey-stick configuration, where the ductus contacts the descending aorta. The oblique/transverse view demonstrates the main pulmonary artery, right pulmonary artery branch, and ductus arteriosus arising from the pulmonary artery. Ductal flow can be detected in most fetuses after 16 weeks' gestation. With increasing gestational age, the ductus increases in diameter and develops a marked curvature, in the configuration of a C or S, which should not be misinterpreted as being abnormal.

Notes

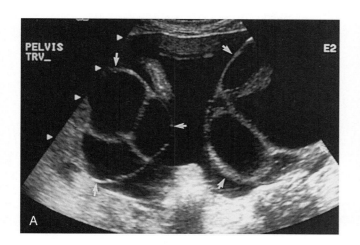

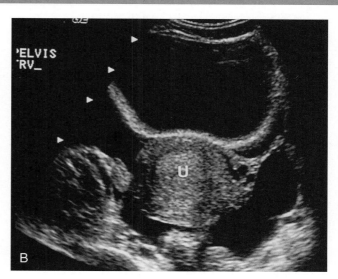

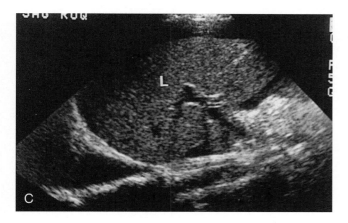

1. Which patients develop the syndrome shown in these transabdominal axial images of the pelvis (Figs. A and B; U = uterus) and sagittal image of the right upper quadrant (Fig. C; L = liver)? What do the arrows denote in Figure B?

2. Who is at increased risk?

3. What are the signs and symptoms?

4. What is the pathophysiology?

Ovarian Hyperstimulation Syndrome

1. Ovarian hyperstimulation caused by ovulation induction or assisted reproduction. Enlarged cystic ovaries

2. Young, lean women with either a "necklace sign" of peripheral ovarian follicles or polycystic ovarian syndrome.

3. Ovarian enlargement and development of ascites.

4. Increased capillary permeability due to large ovarian cysts.

Reference
Berendonk CCM, Van Dop PA, Braat DDM, Merkus JMWM: Ovarian hyperstimulation syndrome: Facts and fallacies. *Obstet Gynecol Surv* 53:439–449, 1998.

Cross-Reference
Ultrasound: THE REQUISITES, pp 391–393.

Comment
Ovarian hyperstimulation syndrome (OHSS) occurs in women undergoing ovulation induction or hyperstimulation for assisted reproduction. Increased capillary permeability due to the large ovarian cysts leads to third spacing, which can result in hypovolemic shock and electrolyte abnormalities. Diagnosis is made by measuring serum estradiol (E_2) levels in a patient with enlargement of the ovaries on ultrasound. Risk factors include a previous history of OHSS as well as the risk of being a young, thin woman. Women with the "necklace sign" of multiple peripheral follicles in the ovary prior to assisted reproduction, or polycystic ovary disease are also at an increased risk.

Luteinization is an integral contributor to the development of OHSS. In particular, the administration of human chorionic gonadotropin increases the risk. Therefore, women who become pregnant are at higher risk for the more severe forms of OHSS.

The ultrasound findings include enlarged ovaries (see Fig. A) and ascites (see Figs. A to C). Unilateral pleural effusion has been described but is rarely as an isolated finding.

Complications in addition to hypovolemic shock (and rarely death) include thromboembolic disease, liver and kidney dysfunction, and acute respiratory distress syndrome. The enlarged ovaries are susceptible to torsion. Treatment is supportive to maintain hemodynamic stability. Transabdominal or transvaginal ultrasound-guided paracentesis has been shown to be an effective treatment. Whereas mild forms can be managed on an outpatient basis, severe OHSS requires hospitalization and even monitoring in an intensive care unit.

Notes

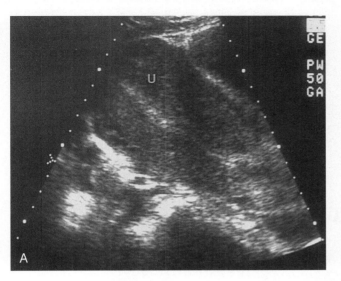

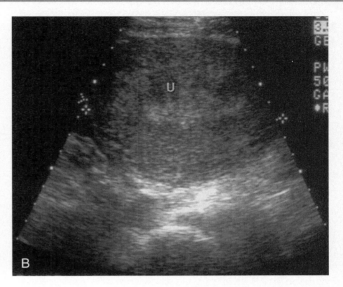

1. This woman, who had a vaginal delivery 2 weeks earlier, presents for an ultrasound (US) examination. She has a fever and pain on abdominal palpation of the uterine fundus (Figs. A and B). Figure A is a sagittal image, and Figure B is an axial image of the uterus (U = uterus). In this case, are there any US findings to suggest the diagnosis of a uterine infection (endometritis or endomyometritis)?

2. Which mode of delivery carries a higher risk of postpartum uterine infection?

3. Does the detection of small foci of gas within the endometrial canal in a postpartum woman confirm the diagnosis of infection? Does mucopurulent discharge indicate an infection postpartum?

4. What percentage of US studies are normal in the setting of acute infection?

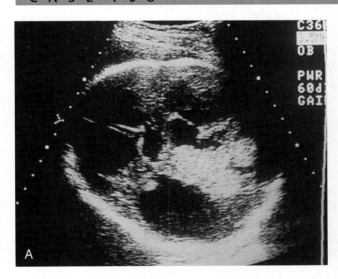

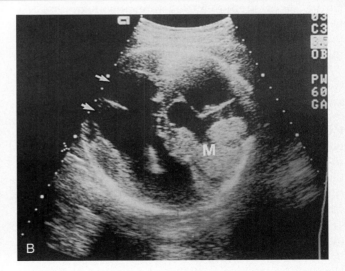

1. In this late second-trimester fetus, the fetal head is markedly enlarged and the parenchyma is greatly distorted (Fig. A). What is the differential diagnosis of this supratentorial parenchymal fetal central nervous system (CNS) abnormality?

2. Where do most fetal CNS tumors arise—supratentorially or infratentorially?

3. What is the most common fetal intracranial neoplasm?

4. How do these patients usually present?

C A S E   1 0 7

Postpartum Endometritis and Endomyometritis

1. There are no specific US findings.

2. Cesarean section.

3. No. No. Mucopurulent discharge can last for 6 weeks postpartum.

4. Up to 50%.

References

Lev-Toaff AS, Baka JJ, Toaff ME, et al: Diagnostic imaging in puerperal febrile morbidity. *Obstet Gynecol* 78:50–55, 1991.

Sweet RL, Ledger WJ: Puerperal infectious morbidity: A two year review. *Am J Obstet Gynecol* 117:1093–1100, 1973.

Wachsberg RH, Kurtz AB: Gas within the endometrial cavity at postpartum US: A normal finding after spontaneous vaginal delivery. *Radiology* 183:4311–422, 1992.

Cross-Reference

Ultrasound: THE REQUISITES, pp 368–374.

Comment

The incidence of endometritis or more severe endomyometritis is much higher following a cesarean section compared with a vaginal delivery: 13% to 39% versus less than 2.7%, respectively. US detects a normal postpartum uterus in up to 50% of women with endometritis or endomyometritis (see Figs. A and B). In this case, the uterus is still prominent in size and has a normally thick endometrial complex (see Fig. A).

When abnormalities are detected, endometrial fluid, debris, and gas may be identified. However, endometrial gas is more commonly a *normal* postpartum finding, even increasing in quantity or appearing over time. A focal abnormality that may contain gas in the anterior uterine wall, however, is suggestive of myometritis. This should not be confused with the normal cesarean scar that is seen as a well-defined oval hyperechoic area or a small (<1.5 cm) subclinical hematoma visualized in or adjacent to the incision in many normal women.

Complications of endomyometritis include wound or pelvic abscess, phlegmon, ovarian vein thrombosis, uterine dehiscence, bacteremia, and death from sepsis. Computed tomography (CT) and magnetic resonance imaging (MRI) are better than US in detecting parametrial inflammation. MRI is particularly useful because of its ability to display in the sagittal plane and is better suited than CT for evaluating the endometrium and anterior myometrium.

Notes

C A S E   1 0 8

Intracranial Teratoma

1. Teratoma, glioblastoma, astrocytoma, lipoma of the corpus callosum, and hemorrhage.

2. Supratentorially.

3. Teratoma.

4. Polyhydramnios and craniomegaly.

References

DiGiovanni LM, Sheikh Z: Prenatal diagnosis, clinical significance and management of fetal intracranial teratoma: A Case report and literature review. *Am J Perinatol* 11:420–422, 1994.

Sherer DM, Onyeije CI: Prenatal ultrasonographic diagnosis of fetal intracranial tumors: A review. *Am J Perinatol* 15:319–328, 1998.

Cross-Reference

Ultrasound: THE REQUISITES, p 225.

Comment

The most common fetal intracranial mass is a supratentorial teratoma. Although it is usually histologically benign, the potential complications from mass effect and high-output cardiac failure yield a very poor prognosis; most of the neonates die soon after birth. These patients often present with polyhydramnios, and the diagnosis is usually made after 20 weeks' gestation. Once detected, the goal is to minimize maternal morbidity at delivery, because the neonatal prognosis is dismal. Decompression of any cystic portions by cephalocentesis may aid in delivery; cesarean section is often required owing to the large circumference of the head.

On ultrasound, an intracranial solid hyperechoic and cystic mass is seen with secondary hydrocephalus (Fig. B, a slightly different projection from Fig. A; M = mass; arrows = dilated lateral ventricles). The head is often enlarged. Such findings are characteristic of a teratoma. Calcification may be present. Polyhydramnios develops, and hydrops with high-output heart failure may also occur.

Other solid CNS tumors are much less common but include glioblastoma and astrocytoma, choroid plexus papilloma (intraventricular with increased cerebrospinal fluid), and medulloblastoma (infratentorial). A parenchymal hemorrhage can appear as a solid, hyperechoic mass. Non-neoplastic causes of a CNS solid mass include heterotopia and hemimegalencephaly. A corpus callosum lipoma is usually midline with variable degrees of agenesis of the corpus callosum as well as additional associated malformations (e.g., encephalocele or meningomyelocele, hypertelorism, median clefting). Conditions that mimic a cystic mass include porencephaly, hydranencephaly, and holoprosencephaly, all of which can be distinguished by findings specific to these entities.

Notes

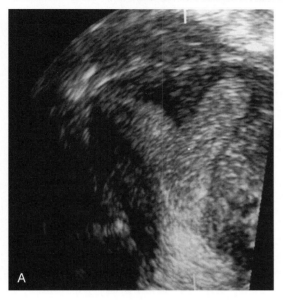

A

1. What is shown on this coronal transvaginal three-dimensional (3-D) reconstructed image of the uterus (Fig. A)?

2. What is the most common congenital uterine anomaly?

3. What is the embryologic precursor of the uterus? Is this the precursor of the vagina as well?

4. What organ system anomaly is associated?

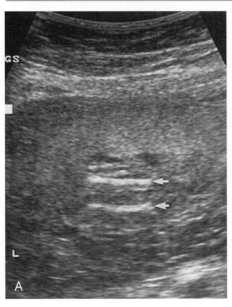

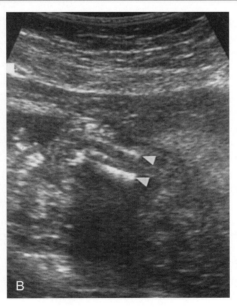

A

B

1. In this third-trimester fetus, which is small-for-dates, transabdominal ultrasound demonstrates the thighs (Fig. A; arrows = femurs) and the lower legs and feet (Fig. B; arrowheads = lower tibias). Is the amount of amniotic fluid normal? What is the differential diagnosis for this unusual configuration that also involved the sacrum?

2. Which is associated with renal agenesis?

3. Which is associated with a two-vessel cord?

4. Which vascular anomaly is associated with sirenomelia?

Congenital Uterine Anomalies

1. Septate uterus.

2. Bicornuate uterus.

3. Müllerian or paramesonephric ducts. No; only the upper two thirds of the vagina.

4. Genitourinary.

Acknowledgment
Figure for Case 109 courtesy of Beryl Benacerraf, MD.

Reference
Pellerito JS, McCarthy SM, Doyle MB, et al: Diagnosis of uterine anomalies: Relative accuracy of MR imaging, endovaginal sonography and hysterosalpingography. *Radiology* 183:795–800, 1992.

Cross-Reference
Ultrasound: THE REQUISITES, p 365.

Comment
The uterus and proximal two thirds of the vagina arise embryologically from the müllerian or paramesonephric ducts. Uterine anomalies are classified into six forms. Class I includes forms of hypoplasia. The unicornuate uterus is class II. Class III is the uterus didelphys. A septate uterus is class IV, and the bicornuate uterus is class V. The congenital anomalies that result from maternal exposure to diethylstilbestrol (DES) during pregnancy constitute class VI.

Because this is also the embryologic precursor of the genitourinary system, renal anomalies are present in 25% of cases. and include renal agenesis, ectopia, malrotation, fusion, and duplication.

Comparative studies have shown that magnetic resonance imaging (MRI) is a more sensitive and accurate modality than transvaginal ultrasound (US) or a hysterosalpingogram for the detection and classification of uterine anomalies. Even for distinguishing a septate uterus, MRI and transvaginal US are very accurate and noninvasive. Recently, 3-D US has been shown to improve the accuracy for detection and differentiation of uterine anomalies, compared with two-dimensional transvaginal imaging. One study showed that the accuracy was comparable with a hysterosalpingography; in addition, 3-D US can distinguish a bicornuate uterus from a septate uterus, which is one limitation of hysterosalpingography.

A septate uterus is distinguished from a bicornuate uterus on transvaginal US and MRI by demonstrating that the fundus is convex, flat, or indented no more than 1 cm (see Fig. A). In addition, the superior portion of the septum is similar in echogenicity (US) or signal intensity (MRI) to myometrial muscle. The inferior portion is fibrous and hypoechoic on US or decreased signal intensity on MRI. A bicornuate uterus has divergent uterine horns and a fundal cleft greater than 1 cm.

Notes

Sirenomelia

1. No; oligohydramnios is present. The differential possibilities are sirenomelia versus caudal regression syndrome.

2. Sirenomelia.

3. Sirenomelia.

4. An aberrant single umbilical artery from the aorta, with distal aortic atresia.

References
Sepulveda W, Romero R, Pryde PG, et al:. Prenatal diagnosis of sirenomelus with color Doppler ultrasonography. *Am J Obstet Gynecol* 170:1377–1379, 1994.

Twickler D, Budorick N, Pretorius D, et al: Caudal regression versus sirenomelia: Sonographic clues. *J Ultrasound Med* 12:323–330, 1993.

Cross-Reference
Ultrasound: THE REQUISITES, p 233.

Comment
Originally believed to be part of a spectrum of anomalies, caudal regression syndrome and sirenomelia have been subsequently shown to have different pathophysiologies and pathologic findings. Caudal regression syndrome occurs in fetuses of diabetic mothers and consists of sacral agenesis and varying degrees of lower spine vertebral body agenesis as well as lower limb hypoplasia. Both kidneys are present, but the bladder and collecting systems may be dilated. An imperforate anus is associated. The volume of amniotic fluid is normal to increased.

Sirenomelia (see Figs. A and B) is a rare lethal malformation with variable degrees of agenesis of the spine and pelvis as well as a single or fused lower extremity. The images here demonstrate the fused lower extremities (see Fig. A, arrows, and Fig. B, arrowheads). The etiology is believed to be a vascular steal of the lower extremity owing to an aberrant single umbilical artery from the aorta and distal aortic atresia. Renal agenesis results in marked oligohydramnios. Note the marked decrease in amniotic fluid in Figures A and B. As a result, the diagnosis may be difficult with prenatal ultrasound. An imperforate anus is also associated with this syndrome.

Color Doppler imaging can assist in the diagnosis of sirenomelia by demonstrating the large single umbilical artery from the aorta to the umbilical cord.

Notes

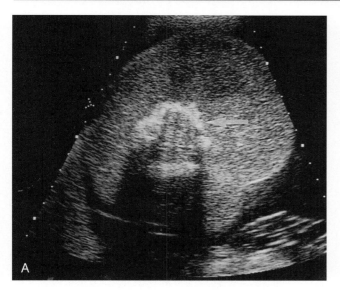

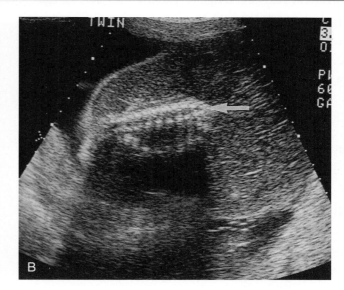

1. In this third-trimester twin pregnancy, one of the twins appears normal. The other has the appearance shown in these two images (Figs. A and B). Figure A is an axial image of the lower chest, and Figure B is a long axis image of the chest and abdomen. The arrow indicates the thoracolumbar spine. What is the diagnosis?

2. What type of twin pregnancy is this?

3. What pathologic abnormality leads to this condition?

4. What is the prognosis for the normal twin?

Acardiac Twin

1. Acardiac twin (acardiac monster).

2. Monochorionic.

3. Abnormal intraplacental arterial-to-arterial and intraplacental venous-to-venous anastomoses.

4. Variable.

References

Fouron J-C, Leduc L, Grigon A, et al: Importance of meticulous ultrasonographic investigation of the acardiac twin. *J Ultrasound Med* 13:1001–1004, 1994.

Hecher K, Ville Y, Nicolaides KH: Color Doppler ultrasonography in the identification of communicating vessels in twin-twin transfusion syndrome and acardiac twins. *J Ultrasound Med* 14:37–40, 1995.

Cross-Reference

Ultrasound: THE REQUISITES, pp 349–351.

Comment

Acardiac twinning is a rare anomaly that arises in twin gestations that share a placenta (monochorionic). Similar to the twin-twin transfusion syndrome, intraplacental vascular anastomoses result in shunting of blood between the normal twin and the acardiac fetus. Unlike the twin-twin transfusion with arteriovenous anastomoses, the connections in this syndrome are different—arterial-arterial and venous-venous. The acardiac fetus is a large dependent mass, which places a large cardiovascular burden on the normal twin. The cardiovascular overload can be fatal.

Ultrasound demonstrates one normal fetus and a large amorphous perfused tissue mass (see Figs. A and B). Limbs may be present, but the mass is usually acephalic. With time, the acardiac twin grows larger than the normal twin, thus creating a large cardiovascular burden in the third trimester. The normal twin develops heart failure and polyhydramnios. Reversal of umbilical artery blood flow is usually present. Reports in the literature have described identification of the communicating intraplacental vessels with color Doppler imaging.

Treatment begins with systemic administration of digitalis. More aggressive treatment options include induction of intravascular thrombosis by injection of substances, selective cesarean delivery, uterotomy, and ligation of the umbilical cord.

Notes

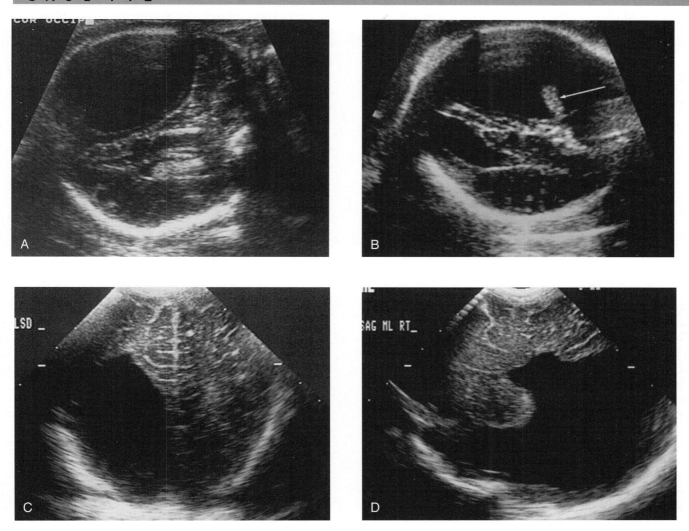

1. What abnormality is seen in these axial images of a third-trimester fetal brain (Figs. A and B)?

2. What is the antenatal differential diagnosis of a nonhydrocephalic cystic central nervous system (CNS) lesion?

3. Which of these communicate with the ventricle?

4. What are three causes of porencephaly?

Porencephaly

1. A cystic lesion replacing a normal brain with associated ventricular dilatation.

2. Arachnoid cyst, porencephalic cyst, hydranencephaly, holoprosencephaly (dorsal cyst) schizencephaly, absent corpus callosum with an interhemispheric cyst, Dandy-Walker malformation, vein of Galen malformation, and teratoma.

3. Porencephaly, dorsal cyst of holoprosencephaly, Dandy-Walker malformation, and schizencephaly.

4. Periventricular leukomalacia, hemorrhage, and infarct.

References

McGahan JP, Ellis W, Lindfors KK, et al: Congenital cerebrospinal fluid-containing intracranial abnormalities: A sonographic classification. *J Clin Ultrasound* 16:531–544, 1988.

Meizner I, Elchalal U: Prenatal sonographic diagnosis of anterior fossa porencephaly. *J Clin Ultrasound* 24:96–99, 1996.

Cross-Reference

Ultrasound: THE REQUISITES, p 225.

Comment

Various congenital disorders can cause cystic brain lesions in the fetus. Determining the cause requires a careful ultrasound examination of the cystic abnormality and the remainder of the brain. In some cases, when the definitive diagnosis cannot be made by ultrasound; magnetic resonance imaging is often helpful.

This case of a large cystic lesion in the brain parenchyma (see Fig. A) with a dilated lateral ventricle (see Fig. B) is an example of porencephaly. The postnatal images above (Figs. C coronal and D sagittal) show a large cyst replacing much of the right side of the neonatal brain. Porencephaly is defined as a cystic parenchymal lesion that communicates with the ventricular system. Potential causes include brain ischemia, hemorrhage, cortical venous thrombosis or vein of Galen thrombosis, infection (e.g., varicella), and periventricular leukomalacia. A pertinent example of an ischemic etiology is the porencephaly detected in early hydranencephaly, or "hydranencephaly in evolution." In these cases, the infarcted parenchyma is replaced by cystic lesions. The porencephalic cyst enlarges with time and can even bulge through the fontanelles, due to cerebrospinal fluid (CSF) excretion by the choroid plexus. With time, the entire cerebral cortex may become replaced by fluid, with only the brainstem and some occipital lobe remaining.

The differential diagnosis of congenital cystic lesions include an arachnoid cyst and the interhemispheric cyst seen with agenesis of the corpus callosum. Open lip schizencephaly may present as a fluid-filled structure representing the connection between the ventricle and CSF surrounding the cerebral cortex. Holoprosencephaly can present with a dorsal cyst that connects to the ventricle, and the Dandy-Walker malformation consists of a large cyst connected to the fourth ventricle. A congenital teratoma can have cystic components but with vascularized solid tissue.

Notes

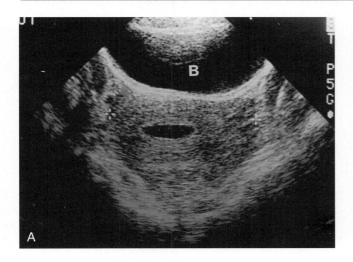

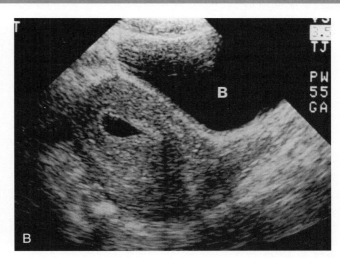

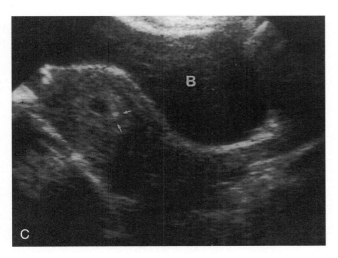

1. Patient A is a young woman who presents with pain for a pelvic ultrasound examination study (Figs. A and B). Figure A is a transabdominal sagittal view, and Figure B is an axial view of the uterus. B = bladder. What is the most likely diagnosis of the intrauterine finding if the pregnancy test result is positive? What is the most likely diagnosis if the pregnancy test result is negative?

2. Patient B is a 23-year-old woman with a transabdominal midline ultrasound image of the uterus (Fig. C; B = bladder). Can you make a definitive diagnosis of this intrauterine finding and, if so, for what reason?

3. Is there a certain mean gestational sac size above which an embryo is expected to be identified both transabdominally and transvaginally?

4. What are the causes of endometritis?

Endometritis

1. With a positive result on a pregnancy test, this is either a normal early intrauterine pregnancy or a pseudogestational sac of an ectopic pregnancy. If the pregnancy test result is negative, endometritis or, less commonly, blood is present.

2. Figure C shows that the double decidual sac (DDS) sign is present (arrows). This strongly indicates a normal intrauterine early pregnancy.

3. Yes; 25 mm by transabdominal scanning and 18 mm by transvaginal scanning.

4. Pelvic inflammatory disease, postpartum, postinstrumentation, and intrauterine device.

References

Neiberg DA, Laing FC, Filly RA, et al: Ultrasonographic differentiation of the gestational sac of early intrauterine pregnancy from the pseudogestational sac of ectopic pregnancy. *Radiology* 146:755–761, 1983.

Pennell RG, Needleman L, Pajak T, et al: Prospective comparison of vaginal and abdominal sonography in normal early pregnancy. J *Ultrasound Med* 10:63–69, 1991.

Cross-Reference

Ultrasound: THE REQUISITES, pp 368–374.

Comment

In a normally menstruating woman, the evaluation of the pelvis must be combined with an accurate menstrual history and pregnancy test. In case A (see Figs. A and B), the uterus has a midline collection. Close analysis shows that it does not have all of the typical properties of a normal intrauterine gestational sac. This collection has a thin hyperechoic rim, is slightly angulated, and has no an intrauterine echoes to suggest an intrauterine pregnancy. In addition, the sac does not have a double decidual sac (DDS) sign, shown in the normal early pregnancy of patient B (see Fig. C, arrows). The DDS sign is caused by the enlarging intrauterine sac impinging on the endometrial canal. The hypoechoic space seen in between two hyperechoic layers is the closed canal. This is detected in more than 95% of normal pregnancies. Failure to see the DDS sign, in a woman who is pregnant, can still be infrequently seen in a normal pregnancy but is much more common in a spontaneous incomplete abortion (miscarriage) or an intrauterine pseudogestational sac, which is seen when there is a collection of endometrial fluid or endometrial hypertrophy under the hormonal influence of an ectopic pregnancy.

In patient A, the pregnancy test result is negative. Presentation with fever should suggest endometritis, especially if the pelvic examination detects a tender or painful uterus. Endometritis, an infection of the endometrial canal, is seen in the puerperium (postpartum) period and post instrumentation (e.g., dilatation and curettage). An intrauterine device predisposed to endometritis. Pelvic inflammatory disease (whether microbacterial or venereal) causes an ascending infection through the vagina, which if left untreated will infect the uterus and then the fallopian tubes and adnexa. These infections, which may spread into the pelvis, can cause peritoneal signs and very infrequently present with right flank and even perihepatic pain owing to an ascending infection.

Notes

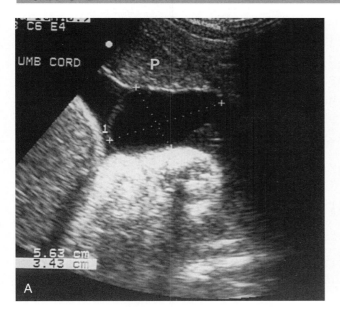

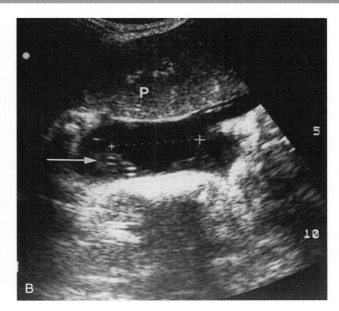

1. What is the differential diagnosis of the cystic abnormality (depicted by + 's and dotted lines) arising from the umbilical cord (arrow) in this third-trimester fetus (Figs. A and B; P = placenta)?

2. Which specific genitourinary anomaly is associated with an allantoic cyst?

3. On which end of the cord are allantoic duct remnants or omphalomesenteric duct remnants usually found?

4. What embryologic arrangement could potentially aid in distinguishing an allantoic duct cyst from an omphalomesenteric duct cyst?

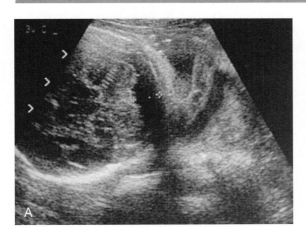

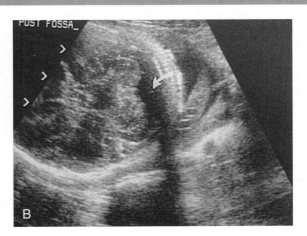

1. What is the normal size range of this anechoic structure (+ 's) within the fetal head (Fig. A)?

2. In this case, this structure measures 15 mm. What is the significance if this structure is enlarged, yet an isolated finding on a prenatal sonogram?

3. With which anomalies is enlargement associated?

4. What does the presence of linear echoes (curved arrow) within this structure suggest in the setting of enlargement (Fig. B)?

Umbilical Cord Cyst

1. True umbilical cord cysts (including allantoic or omphalomesenteric cysts), Wharton's jelly cyst, umbilical cord hematoma or hemangioma, and umbilical vessel dilatation.

2. A patent urachus.

3. The fetal end.

4. Allantoic duct remnants are surrounded by umbilical vessels, and are located in the center of the cord. Omphalomesenteric duct cysts arise eccentrically.

References

Dudiak CM, Salomon CG, Posniak HV, et al: Sonography of the umbilical cord. *Radiographics* 15:1035–1050, 1995.

Kalter CS, Williams MC, Vaughn V, Spellacy WN: Sonographic diagnosis of a large umbilical cord pseudocyst. *J Ultrasound Med* 13:487–489, 1994.

Cross-Reference

Ultrasound: THE REQUISITES, pp 313–315.

Comment

Cystic masses of the umbilical cord may be true cysts (allantoic duct or omphalomesenteric duct remnants), dilated vasculature, or pseudocysts (e.g., Wharton's Jelly cysts). Once a cystic mass is detected, it is difficult to determine the exact etiology with antenatal ultrasound. Color Doppler imaging should be used to determine if the vessels of the cord are compressed or thrombosed and to exclude a vascular anomaly as the cause of the cyst. Follow-up scans should be performed throughout the gestation.

Cysts that arise from either allantoic or omphalomesenteric ducts can be associated with genitourinary (GU) and gastrointestinal (GI) anomalies. Specific associations include a bowel or GU obstruction, hernia, omphalocele, and patent urachus. The association with patent urachus is essential to recognize to avoid the complication of transection of the urachus when cutting the umbilical cord, particularly if the cyst arises close to the anterior abdominal wall of the fetus.

Omphalomesenteric duct cysts are lined with epithelium that can differentiate into gastric epithelia and possibly secrete acid. Ulceration can occur, resulting in a fetal hemorrhage.

Pseudocysts are collections of liquefied Wharton's jelly which may resolve, but have also been reported in association with trisomy 18 and trisomy 13.

Notes

Large Cisterna Magna

1. 2 to 10 mm.

2. Probably a normal variant.

3. Dandy-Walker malformation, trisomy 18.

4. A normal variant.

References

Haimovici JA, Doubilet PM, Benson CB, Frates MC: Clinical significance of isolated enlargement of the cisterna magna (>10 mm) on prenatal sonography. *J Ultrasound Med* 16:731–734, 1997.

Pretorius DH, Kallman CE, Grafe MR, et al: Linear echos in the fetal cisterna magna. *J Ultrasound Med* 11:125–128, 1992.

Cross-Reference

Ultrasound: THE REQUISITES, pp 219–221.

Comment

The routine obstetric ultrasound of the fetal head includes an evaluation of the posterior fossa: the cerebellum and cisterna magna, which is the fluid-filled structure directly posterior to the cerebellum. The posterior fossa should be imaged in an axial plane through the thalami, with 10 to 15 degrees of angulation. Proper technique is essential, because more coronal imaging can create a false enlargement of the cisterna magna, which should range in anteroposterior diameter from 2 to 10 mm. The normal cisterna magna usually has linear echoes that run perpendicular to the occipital bone, particularly if the cisterna magna measures more than 3 mm. These echoes are believed to represent dural folds, the falx cerebelli, or subarachnoid septa.

Effacement or enlargement of the cisterna magna raises concern for associated anomalies, particularly if the cerebellum is abnormal. Effacement suggests a Chiari II malformation; the hindbrain defect includes a malformed (banana shaped) cerebellum. Enlargement of the cisterna magna with cerebellar vermian agenesis indicates a Dandy-Walker malformation. Cisterna magna enlargement has also been associated with trisomy 18, but these fetuses usually have either cerebellar or other additional structural anomalies.

This case demonstrates a normal variant enlargement of the cisterna magna. The cerebellum and brain must be normal to classify this finding as a normal variant, and there can be no other structural anomalies. One series reported that 15 cases of isolated enlargement of the cisterna magna (from 11 to 19 mm) were associated with a normal neonatal outcome. The enlargement associated with a Dandy Walker malformation is more commonly anechoic, although this is not an absolute rule.

Notes

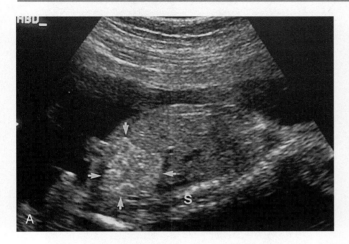

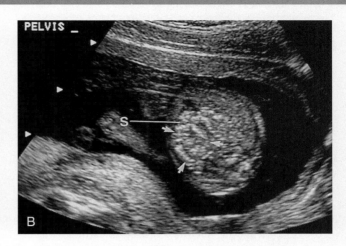

1. In two 20-week fetal studies, arrows outline the lower abdominal areas. Which of these areas is abnormal? Figure A shows the right parasagittal image of the body. Figure B is the axial image of the fetal lower abdomen. S = the fetal spine.

2. What degree of bowel echogenicity is considered abnormal?

3. Are there associated abnormalities?

4. True or false: echogenic bowel that resolves in the third trimester has no clinical significance?

Echogenic Bowel

1. Figure A is abnormal.

2. If equal to or more echogenic (hyperechoic) than bone such as the spine or iliac crests.

3. Yes.

4. False.

References

Grignon A, Dubois J, Ouellet MC, et al: Echogenic dilated bowel loops before 21 weeks' gestation: A new entity. *AJR Am J Roentgenol* 168:833–837, 1997.

Nyberg DA, Dubinsky T, Resta RG, et al: Echogenic fetal bowel during the second trimester: Clinical importance. *Radiology* 188:527–531, 1993.

Paulson EK, Hertzberg BS. Hyperechoic meconium in the third trimester fetus: An uncommon normal variant. *J Ultrasound Med* 10:677–680, 1991.

Cross-Reference

Ultrasound: THE REQUISITES, pp 262–265.

Comment

Echogenic fetal bowel is probably a combination of mesentery and small bowel. The cause of the increased echogenicity has been hypothesized to be decreased fluid content of the meconium. It is important, however, to recognize that meconium can be echogenic in the third trimester, particularly late in the gestation, as a normal variant.

Echogenic bowel can occur in any part of the abdomen but is most common in the right lower quadrant. The prognosis depends on the other concomitant abnormalities: in utero infection, cystic fibrosis, meconium ileus, and chromosomal anomalies, most commonly Down syndrome but also trisomy 18, trisomy 13, and triploidy. Because of the associated anomalies, the prognosis must remain guarded even if the echogenic bowel resolves.

All echogenic bowel is not abnormal. To be considered abnormal, the area is expected to have an echogenicity (brightness) greater than bone such as the spine or iliac crests. The echogenic bowel is expected to be larger than 4 cm and to often exhibit a mass effect on adjacent structures. Figure A is abnormal, in a fetus with Down syndrome, and meets the aforementioned criteria. Figure B is normal and has an area that is less echogenic and smaller.

Echogenic dilated bowel loops (EDBL) (Fig. C; arrows) is a distinct abnormality—either an isolated (one quadrant) or diffuse (more than one quadrant) gastrointestinal abnormality. It is detected in the second trimester as bowel 2 to 10 mm in diameter with an echogenic wall. In almost all cases, the finding resolves

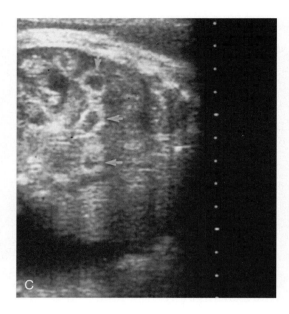

by the third trimester. As an isolated finding, it is benign. However, the complex form has a worse outcome because of associated anomalies. Such abnormalities include gastroschisis, meconium peritonitis, VATER (imperforate anus), malrotation, and bowel atresia. The etiology is believed to be bowel obstruction and is confirmed by decreased amniotic fluid disaccharidase activity.

Detection of either of these findings in the second trimester warrants prenatal and postnatal follow-up. A careful search for associated anomalies is imperative.

Notes

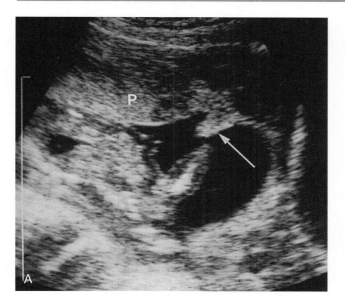
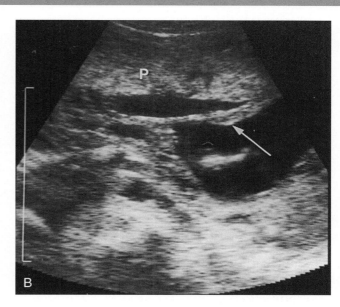

1. In this third-trimester pregnancy, what is the name of this outpouching (arrow) at the edge of the placenta (P) into the amniotic fluid (Fig. A)?

2. What complications have been associated?

3. Is ultrasound a sensitive screening tool to detect this placental abnormality?

4. What is the diagnosis and differential diagnosis of this large soft tissue band (arrow) in another third-trimester pregnancy (Fig. B; P = placenta)?

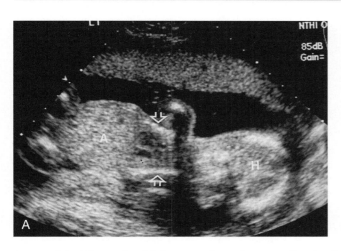
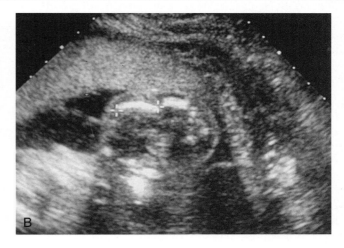

1. In this 20-week-old fetus, what abnormality is shown in the coronal image of the fetus (Fig. A; H = head, A = abdomen; open arrows = chest) and the long axis image of one of its femurs (Fig. B; +'s = femoral shaft)? What is the likely diagnosis?

2. Which calvarial anomaly is frequently described with this disorder?

3. What is the outcome?

4. How many spine ossification centers are typically present at each vertebral level, and what is the significance?

Circumvallate Placenta (Placenta Extrachorialis)

1. Circumvallate placenta.

2. Low birthweight, premature labor, placental abruption, intrauterine growth retardation, fetal anomalies, and perinatal death.

3. No.

4. Amniotic shelf (or amniotic sheet). The differential diagnosis is a circumvallate placenta and an amniotic band.

References

Harris RD, Wells WA, Black WC, et al: Accuracy of prenatal sonography for detecting circumvallate placenta. *AJR Am J Roentgenol* 168:1602–1608, 1997.

McCarthy J, Thurmond AS, Jones MK, et al: Circumvallate placenta: Sonographic diagnosis. *J Ultrasound Med* 14:21–26, 1995.

Cross-Reference

Ultrasound: THE REQUISITES, p 313.

Comment

Circumvallate placenta or placenta extrachorialis is not an uncommon disorder. Complete circumvallate placenta occurs in 1% of pregnancies; partial circumvallate placenta is estimated to occur 10 to 20 times more commonly. It results from a mismatch in growth at the placental margin. In typical placentation, there is a smooth transition from the parenchymal villous chorion to the membranous chorion. In circumvallate placenta, either partial or complete, the parenchymal villous chorion overgrows and bulges into the amniotic fluid. This leaves villous tissue of the chorionic frondosum that is not completely covered by the amniochorionic membrane, hence the term placenta extrachorialis. As a result, the parenchymal villous chorionic tissue bulges out peripherally, and the edge of the placenta develops a rolled appearance (see Fig. A).

Amniotic shelves or sheets, (see Fig. B) thought to be due to synechiae covered by amniochorionic membrane, are usually larger but otherwise similar in appearance to a circumvallate placenta.

The clinical significance of a circumvallate placenta is uncertain. It has been associated with low birthweight, prematurity, intrauterine growth retardation, placental abruption, and perinatal death. In addition, congenital anomalies may be present, although the exact etiology of this finding is uncertain. Unfortunately, ultrasound is neither sensitive nor specific for diagnosis, as shown by one study done by experienced sonologists.

Notes

Thanatophoric Dysplasia (Thanatophoric Dwarfism)

1. Narrow thorax (see Fig. A), shortened bowed long bone (see Fig. B). Thanatophoric dysplasia or dwarfism.

2. Cloverleaf skull.

3. Lethal.

4. Three ossification centers; distinguishes from achondrogenesis, which often has less.

Acknowledgment

Figure for Case 118 courtesy of Beryl Benacerraf, MD.

References

Bowerman RA: Anomalies of the fetal skeleton: Sonographic findings. *AJR Am J Roentgenol* 164:973–979, 1995.

Pretorius DH, Rumack CM, Manc-Johnson ML, et al: Specific skeletal dysplasias in utero: Sonographic diagnosis. *Radiology* 159:237–242, 1986.

Cross-Reference

Ultrasound: THE REQUISITES, pp 301–302.

Comment

Thanatophoric dysplasia or dwarfism is a lethal dwarfism with many characteristic findings. The differential diagnosis of short-limbed dwarfism includes achondrogenesis, campomelic dwarfism, homozygous achondroplasia, severe hypophosphatasia, and severe osteogenesis imperfecta.

The features of thanatophoric dysplasia common to the other lethal dysplasias include a narrow thorax due to short ribs (see Fig. A) and shortened bowed long bones (see Fig. B). Characteristic findings that aid in distinguishing thanatophoric dysplasia include macrocephaly with frontal bossing and hydrocephalus. A cloverleaf skull, also known as "kleeblattschädel," is a classic finding but is present in only 14% of cases. The "telephone receiver" configuration of the shortened, bowed long bones is also characteristic for this disorder (see Fig. B). The skin may be thickened, and vertebral bodies flattened (platyspondyly). However, the spine ossification is normal.

The narrowed chest results in pulmonary hypoplasia, contributing to the high mortality. Polyhydramnios and hydrops often develop in utero. The presence of kleeblattschädel is important, because this may represent a subtype of thanatophoric dysplasia that is transmitted as an autosomal recessive trait with a risk of recurrence of 25%.

Notes

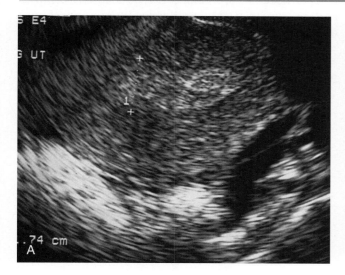

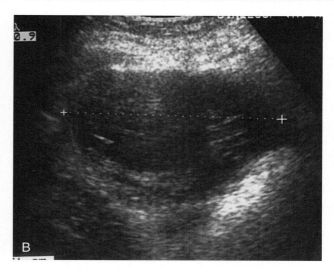

1. This 50-year-old woman presents with abnormal vaginal bleeding and lower abdominal pain. A transvaginal pelvic study of the uterus (Fig. A, sagittal midline image; +'s = the 17-mm endometrial thickness) and right ovary (Fig. B, axial/coronal image; +'s = 5.1 cm in the longest axis) was performed. What are the findings, and what is the most likely diagnosis?

2. Which subtype of this tumor is more likely to be malignant?

3. What is a Call-Exner body?

4. Which subtype is more likely to have an associated endometrial cancer?

Sex Cord Stromal (Granulosa Stromal Cell) Tumor

1. Solid ovarian mass and increased endometrial thickening. Diagnosis: a sex cord stromal tumor.

2. Granulosa stromal cell type.

3. Call-Exner bodies are the microfollicular and macrofollicular patterns (rosette-like) that are seen with granulosa cells when viewed cytologically.

4. Thecoma.

References

Cronje HS, Niemand I, Bam RH, Woodruff JD: Review of the granulosa-theca cell tumors from the Emil Novak Ovarian Tumor Registry. *Am J Obstet Gynecol* 180:323–327, 1999.

Morikawa K, Hatabu H, Togashi K, et al: Granulosa cell tumor of the ovary: MR findings. *J Comput Assist Tomogr* 21:1001–1004, 1997.

Segal R, DePetrillo AD, Thomas G: Clinical review of adult granulosa cell tumors of the ovary. *Gynecol Oncol* 56:338–344, 1995.

Cross-Reference
Ultrasound: THE REQUISITES, pp 407–413.

Comment
The sex cord stromal tumors represent an uncommon subset of ovarian neoplasms. The subtypes include the granulosa-stromal cell, thecoma-fibroma, and Sertoli-Leydig cell tumors. The first two types can secrete estrogens, whereas the latter may secrete androgenic hormones and cause virilization.

Granulosa stromal cell tumors and thecomas, which produce estrogen, can result in endometrial hyperplasia or endometrial cancer. This case demonstrates an ovarian granulosa cell tumor (see Fig. B) with associated endometrial hyperplasia (see Fig. A). Thecomas are more commonly estrogenic and have a higher incidence of associated endometrial abnormality than do granulosa cell stromal tumors. However, the granulosa cell tumor is prone to rupture and is more likely to be malignant, with a propensity for late recurrences.

Histologically, Call-Exner bodies may be seen; these are macrofollicles or microfollicles. Gross pathologic studies have shown that these tumors are often large and that they have a mean size of 10 cm. Theca cell tumors are more commonly solid. Granulosa cell tumors can be solid, multicystic, or both. Either type can cause ovarian torsion. In many cases, hemorrhage is detected within the mass, which may be seen on ultrasound or magnetic resonance imaging (MRI). Ultrasound and MRI will also reveal any associated uterine enlargement and endometrial thickening that results from the hormonal secretion.

The detection of a multicystic or solid ovarian mass and endometrial thickening via ultrasound should prompt consideration of one of these sex cord stromal tumors.

Notes

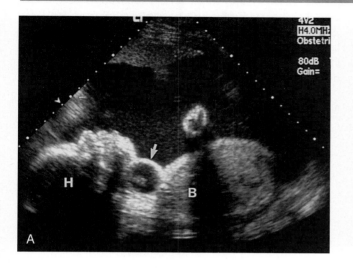

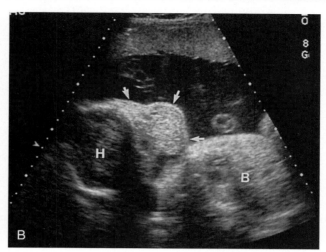

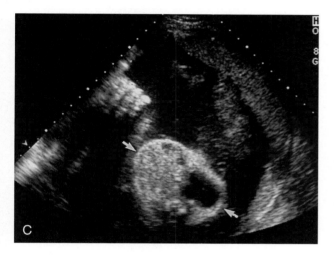

1. What is the most likely diagnosis and differential diagnosis for the neck abnormality (arrows) noted in this early third-trimester fetus (Figs. A to C, sagittal, coronal, axial, respectively; H = head; B = body)?

2. How does the location aid in narrowing the differential?

3. What abnormality of amniotic fluid can be seen with a cervical teratoma (see Figs. A to C)?

4. What ultrasound finding would aid in distinguishing a teratoma from a cystic hygroma?

Cervical Teratoma

1. Cervical teratoma is the most likely diagnosis. The differential diagnoses are cystic hygroma, fetal goiter, thyroglossal duct cyst or branchial cleft cyst, and congenital neuroblastoma.

2. Teratomas, thyroglossal duct cyst, and goiter more commonly anterior; branchial cleft cysts are lateral; cystic hygromas are more commonly posterior/lateral (but may occur anteriorly).

3. Polyhydramnios in 20% of cervical teratomas.

4. Calcifications can be seen with teratoma, which can have solid and cystic components; a cystic hygroma is cystic with septations.

References

Kerner B, Flaum E, Mathews H, et al: Cervical teratoma: Prenatal diagnosis and long-term follow-Up. *Prenat Diagn* 18:51–59, 1998.

Tsuda H, Matsumoto M, Yamamoto K, et al: Usefulness of ultrasonography and magnetic resonance imaging for prenatal diagnosis of fetal teratoma of the neck. *J Clin Ultrasound* 24:217–219, 1996.

Cross-Reference

Ultrasound: THE REQUISITES, p 233.

Comment

A fetal neck mass can arise from various locations, which may aid in narrowing the differential diagnosis; however, these rules are not 100%. A cystic hygroma classically arises from the posterior and lateral parts of the neck, but a subtype can arise anteriorly and even extend into the superior mediastinum. Because of their thyroid origin, fetal goiter and thyroglossal duct cysts arise anteriorly. Branchial cleft cysts are generally found in the lateral neck. The cervical teratoma can present in any part of the neck but more commonly is seen anteriorly.

This case demonstrates a large cystic and solid teratoma in the anterior cervical region (see Figs. A to C). Fetal teratomas can arise anywhere in the body; the cervical region is rare (5%). On ultrasound, a cystic and solid mass is seen; calcifications are present in 50% of cases. Because of the solid nature of the mass, the head is often forced into a fixed extended position. Polyhydramnios, as is also present in this case, develops in 20%, due to the inability of the fetus to swallow amniotic fluid. Pathologically, these are usually benign and encapsulated. The α-fetoprotein (AFP) level can be elevated. No associated anomalies are present.

Malignant degeneration of a cervical teratoma in utero is rare. Morbidity and mortality relate to respiratory distress at birth. Prenatal detection is essential for proper delivery and immediate stabilization of the airway. Surgical resection improves mortality from 100% to 23%. Factors associated with a poor prognosis include a large size (>8 cm diameter), rapid growth, invasion of vital structures (e.g., carotid artery, trachea, larynx), or rarely a malignancy.

Notes

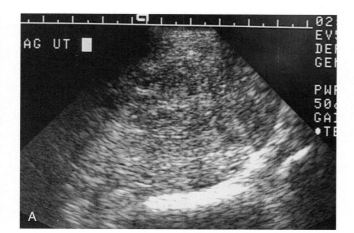

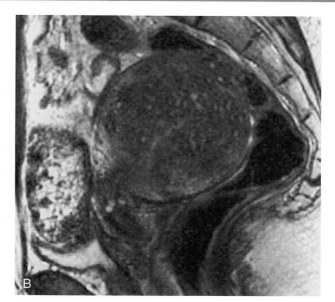

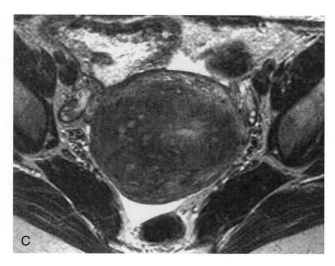

1. What findings are shown in this transvaginal sagittal ultrasound image of the uterus in a 40-year-old woman (Fig. A)? What are the differential possibilities?

2. What are the magnetic resonance imaging (MRI) findings of the uterus in the same patient (Figs. B and C)? Figure B is a T₂-weighted sagittal image, and Figure C is a T₂-weighted axial image.

3. How do women present with adenomyosis?

4. Can this entity present as a mass that mimics a myoma?

Adenomyosis

1. An indistinct junctional zone (between the endometrium and the myometrium), inhomogeneity of the myometrium, and perhaps some myometrial cysts. The differential diagnosis is adenomyosis versus multiple small fibroids.

2. A prominent uterus with thickening of the junctional zone with high signal foci in the myometrium.

3. Menorrhagia, dysmenorrhagia, and uterine enlargement.

4. Yes.

References

Brosens JJ, Barker FC: Adenomyosis: Time for a reappraisal. *Lancet* 341:181–182, 1993.

Reinhold C, McCarthy S, Bret PM, et al: Diffuse adenomyosis: Comparison of endovaginal US and MR imaging with histopathologic correlation. *Radiology* 199:151–158, 1996.

Schnall M: Magnetic resonance evaluation of acquired benign uterine disorders. *Semin Ultrasound CT MR* 15:18–26, 1994.

Cross-Reference

Ultrasound: THE REQUISITES, pp 378–379.

Comment

Adenomyosis is defined as ectopic endometrial glands and stroma in the myometrium. Unlike endometriosis, only 13% of these glandular implants respond to endogenous estrogen and progesterone stimulation. Women present with menorrhagia or dysmenorrhagia and enlargement of the uterus.

This case of adenomyosis demonstrates loss of the discrete junctional zone, which appears heterogeneous (see Fig. A). In most cases, the uterus is enlarged. Detection of irregular, cystic spaces in the myometrium is the finding most specific for adenomyosis on ultrasound. However, several studies have shown findings that can be much more subtle on ultrasound, including loss of the junctional zone, a slight decrease in the echogenicity of the uterus, posterior uterine wall thickening, and displacement of the endometrial lining. A focal region of adenomyosis, called an adenomyoma, can be seen in some cases. This may have a more irregular shape than the characteristic rounded appearance of a leiomyoma.

MRI is at least as sensitive and accurate in making the diagnosis of adenomyosis. On MRI, many of the findings reflect smooth muscle proliferation in reaction to the heterotopic endometrial tissue. The junctional zone is thickened, and a cutoff of 12 mm is used to suggest the diagnosis. Small foci with high signal intensity are seen within the myometrium on T_2-weighted sequences (see Figs. B and C) and sometimes on a T_1-weighted image.

It is important to distinguish focal adenomyosis from a leiomyoma because the treatment is different. MRI is helpful in this role, particularly when subtle ultrasound findings are present and because the appearance of an adenomyoma as a calcified uterine mass, mimicking a myoma on ultrasound, has been reported in the literature. On MRI, the borders of an adenomyoma are irregular, and the presence of the high signal foci in the myometrium on T_2-weighted sequences should aid in the distinction of these two entities.

Notes

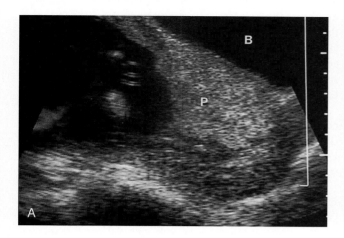

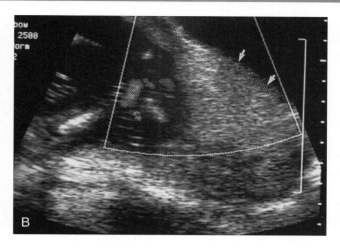

1. In this third-trimester pregnancy, Figure A is a sagittal transabdominal scan of the lower uterine segment (P = placenta; B = urinary bladder). Figure B, a color Doppler image of Figure A, shows flow denoted by arrows. What is the diagnosis, and which three entities comprise its spectrum of abnormality?

2. Name three risk factors.

3. List three potential complications.

4. What are three characteristic ultrasound findings?

Placental Invasion (Accreta, Increta, and Percreta)

1. Placenta percreta. Placental invasion of the uterine wall is categorized as placenta accreta (up to), increta (into), and percreta (through) depending on the depth of myometrial invasion.

2. Risk factors include previous uterine surgery (particularly a cesarean section), a placenta previa, or a history of a retained placenta.

3. Bladder invasion and rupture, uterine infection or wall rupture and uterine inversion.

4. An anterior placenta, ranging from a low-lying previa to a total previa; absence of the normal subplacental anechoic/hypoechoic zone composed of the myometrium and junctional zone; subplacental vascular spaces.

Reference
Hoffman-Tretin JC, Koenigsberg M, Rabin A, et al: Placenta accreta: Additional sonographic observations. *J Ultrasound Med* 1:29–34, 1992.

Cross-Reference
Ultrasound: THE REQUISITES, pp 318–322.

Comment
Placental invasion of the uterine wall is categorized as placenta accreta, percreta, or increta depending on the depth of the myometrial invasion. Myometrial contact by villi without invasion is called accreta. Invasion into the myometrium or through the myometrium with serosal penetration is labeled increta or percreta, respectively. The case shown here demonstrates invasion through the myometrium to the bladder. Villi penetrate into the myometrium due to a deficiency of the decidua basalis, typically caused by prior disruption of the endometrium. At delivery, hemorrhage results because the placenta cannot detach.

The most common predisposing risk factors are placenta previa, previous uterine surgery (cesarean section, myomectomy, or curettage), a history of a retained placenta, or multiparity. If the placenta implants over a site of disrupted endometrium, such as the anterior lower uterine segment of a post-cesarean uterus, the risk of invasion is quite high.

If an invasion is not detected antenatally, patients can present with massive hemorrhage at delivery because the placenta fails to normally detach. The diagnosis can be suggested by recognizing several important ultrasound findings. The placenta is anterior, ranging from low lying to complete previa. Invasion may be reflected by the absence of the normal subplacental anechoic/hypoechoic zone, composed of a junctional zone. This

can be focally or entirely absent. In percreta, extension may involve the bladder wall. Other associated findings include a heterogeneous echotexture of the placenta, the presence of a few or numerous subplacental vascular spaces, and enlargement of parauterine veins. If the subplacental myometrium is only thinned, this could represent a normal finding; however, accreta cannot then be excluded, particularly if risk factors are present.

In this case, Figures A and B show an anterior placenta previa (P), which is invading the bladder wall (B). The abnormal blood vessels are detected by color Doppler imaging. The diagnosis of a placenta percreta was made prior to delivery.

Complications include bladder invasion and rupture, uterine infection, uterine wall rupture, and uterine inversion. Despite attempts to control blood loss with a hysterectomy, patients may still lose substantial quantities of blood. Recently, control of the bleeding with interventional embolization techniques has been attempted to facilitate a hysterectomy with less blood loss.

Notes

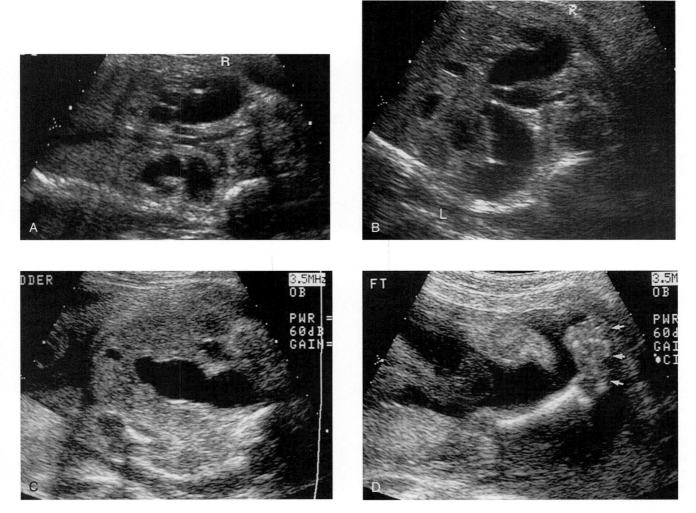

1. What is the differential diagnosis of the third-trimester fetus (Figs. A to C)? Figure A is a coronal image of the kidneys; Figure B is a coronal image of the lower abdomen below the kidneys; and Figure C is an axial image of the pelvis. R = fetal right side; L = fetal left side in Figures A and B.

2. Which occurs more commonly in males?

3. For which condition is vesicoamniotic shunting more appropriate?

4. Which condition has associated musculoskeletal anomalies (Fig. D; arrows point to a fetal foot)?

Prune-Belly Syndrome

1. Prune-belly syndrome, urethral stenosis or agenesis, and posterior urethral valves.

2. Both posterior urethral valves and prune-belly syndrome; posterior urethral valves occur exclusively in males.

3. Posterior urethral valves and urethral agenesis.

4. Prune-belly syndrome.

References

Brinker MR, Palutsis RS, Sarwark JF: The orthopedic manifestations of prune-belly (Eagle-Barrett) syndrome. *J Bone Joint Surg* 77-A:251–257, 1995.

Smith CA, Smith Edwin A, Parrott TS, et al: Voiding function in patients with the prune-belly syndrome after Monfort abdominoplasty. *J Urol* 159:1675–1679, 1998.

Woodard JR: Lesson learned in three decades of managing the prune-belly syndrome (Editorial). *J Urol* 159:1680, 1998.

Cross-Reference

Ultrasound: THE REQUISITES, pp 281, 286–287.

Comment

Prune-belly syndrome is believed by many to be a generalized mesenchymal disorder as opposed to an obstructive uropathy. It is manifested by dilatation of the renal collecting systems, absence or hypoplasia of the abdominal musculature, and cryptorchidism. The absence of normal abdominal muscles results in a wrinkled appearance to the skin of the anterior abdominal wall, and the abdomen is protuberant. Prune-belly syndrome, also known as Eagle-Barrett syndrome, is much more common in males.

On prenatal ultrasound, various forms of dilatation of the pelvicaliceal system and ureters is seen. This case demonstrates bilateral renal pelvicaliceal dilatation (see Fig. A), bilateral ureteral dilatation (see Fig. B), and a thick-walled prominent and unusually shaped urinary bladder (see Fig. C). The anterior abdominal wall abnormality can be difficult to visualize. The differential diagnosis of a bilateral ureteral obstruction includes posterior urethral valves, which occur exclusively in males, and urethral atresia.

Several musculoskeletal anomalies are associated with prune-belly syndrome and can be sought if the diagnosis is suspected on prenatal ultrasound. The most common abnormality is subluxation or dislocation of the hip, which is often resistant to traditional treatment. Scoliosis, chest wall deformity (pectus excavatum), and renal osteodystrophy have also been described in children with prune-belly syndrome. In this case, the fetus had a clubfoot (see Fig. D).

Vesicoamniotic shunting has not necessarily been shown to improve the renal function. Postnatal treatment is directed at reconstruction of the urinary system, orchiopexy, and surgical repair of the anterior abdominal wall. The genitourinary function correlates with bladder function as well. Furthermore, repair of the anterior abdominal wall improves bowel and bladder function.

Notes

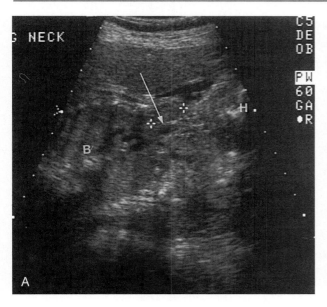

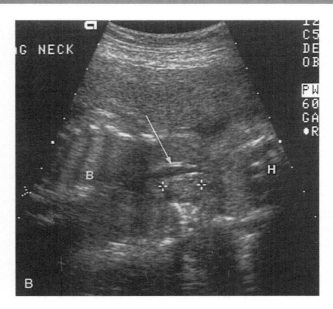

1. What is being measured (+'s) in the neck of these coronal images of a third-trimester fetus (Figs. A and B; H = head)?

2. What is denoted by an arrow in both of these images?

3. What is the usual etiology of this disorder?

4. What are the potential consequences if the disorder is left untreated?

CASE 125

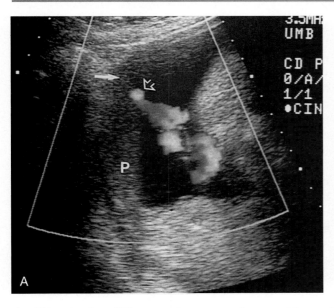

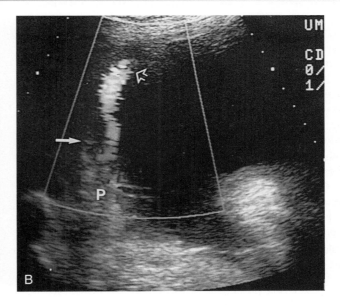

1. What is the difference between the cord insertion in the color Doppler images of the placenta (P) in Figures A and B? Closed arrow = margin of the placenta; open arrow = insertion of the umbilical cord.

2. Are there problems associated with a marginal cord insertion?

3. Is a velamentous cord insertion more common in multiple pregnancies?

4. What are the complications or anomalies associated with velamentous cord insertion?

Fetal Goiter

1. Right and left lobes of an enlarged thyroid.

2. Trachea.

3. Treatment of maternal Graves' disease with propylthiouracil (PTU).

4. Obstruction of the airway or esophagus; hyperextension of the neck. Lower intelligence scores.

Reference

Van Loon AJ, Derksen JTM, Bos AF, Rouwe CW: In utero diagnosis and treatment of fetal goitrous hypothyroidism, caused by maternal use of propylthiouracil. *Prenat Diagn* 15:599-604, 1995.

Cross-Reference

Ultrasound: THE REQUISITES, p 233.

Comment

Enlargement of the fetal thyroid gland may be associated with a hypothyroid or hyperthyroid state. Fetal goiter, demonstrated by these coronal images of the fetal neck, can be detected and followed after treatment with prenatal ultrasound. The differential diagnosis of an anterior neck mass in utero includes teratoma, thyroglossal duct cyst (midline), and branchial cleft cyst, which is usually lateral. Rarely, a cystic hygroma may present anteriorly.

In patients with Graves' disease, the thyroid-stimulating immunoglobulins cross the placenta and cause fetal hyperthyroidism. Despite early neonatal treatment, developmental disorders can result.

Alternatively, fetal hypothyroidism is caused by the transplacental transfer of medications (e.g., PTU) used to treat maternal hyperthyroidism. Agenesis or hypoplasia of the fetal thyroid is an additional cause. Polyhydramnios may be present. The neonate may develop cardiovascular or respiratory abnormalities as well as mental retardation.

Cordocentesis is the only accurate method to determine fetal thyroid hormone levels. Treatment of hyperthyroidism is possible with maternally administered PTU; however, hypothyroidism requires fetal intramuscular, intravascular, or intra-amniotic infusion of thyroxine.

Notes

Velamentous Insertion of the Umbilical Cord

1. Figure A shows a marginal cord insertion. Figure B shows a velamentous cord insertion, an insertion of the umbilical cord into the amniochorionic membranes beyond the placental margin.

2. No.

3. Yes, 10 times more common.

4. Rupture during labor causing fetal exsanguination, preterm delivery, intrauterine growth restriction (IUGR), single umbilical artery anomalies, and other congenital anomalies.

References

Pretorius DH, Chau C, Poelter DM, et al: Placental cord insertion visualization with prenatal ultrasonography. *J Ultrasound Med* 15:585-593, 1996.

Raga F, Ballester MJ, Osborne NG, Bonilla-Musoles F: Role of Color flow Doppler ultrasonography in diagnosing velamentous insertion of the umbilical cord and vasa previa. *J Reprod Med* 40:804-808, 1995.

Cross-Reference

Ultrasound: THE REQUISITES, pp 313-315.

Comment

Marginal cord insertion is defined as peripheral insertion of the cord in the placenta, within 2 cm of the edge. Velamentous insertion is distinguished by aberrant vessels traversing between the amnion and chorion before placental insertion. Velamentous cord insertion occurs in 1.1% of single intrauterine gestations, with a 10 times higher incidence in multiple pregnancies. It is also associated with uterine anomalies and indwelling intrauterine devices (IUDs).

A velamentous insertion carries the risk of several complications. With active labor, a velamentous insertion is not anchored and can tear, resulting in exsanguination. Preterm delivery occurs in 17% of cases. IUGR, single umbilical artery, congenital anomalies, and low Apgar scores have also been reported. A vasa previa caused by a velamentous insertion in front of the presenting part of the fetus may be associated.

Ultrasound studies have reported a 42% sensitivity for detection of an abnormal placental cord insertion, particularly later in the gestation. Nonetheless, this is an important portion of the prenatal sonogram evaluation. The use of color Doppler imaging facilitates visualization of the insertion site.

Notes

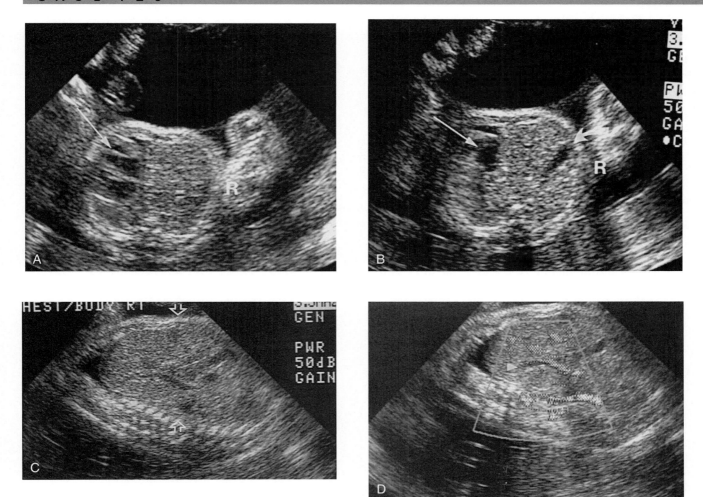

1. In this second-trimester fetus, what is the differential diagnosis for this axial image of the chest (Fig. A; R = the right side of the fetus; arrow = the heart. What is the diagnosis once Figure B is also taken into account? What does the curved arrow denote?

2. In the same case, what does the sagittal image of the right side of the fetal chest show (Fig. C)? Open arrows show the bottom of the chest.

3. In Figure D, the color Doppler image of Figure C, what does the arrowhead point denote?

4. Can the liver herniate into a left-sided diaphragmatic hernia?

Congenital Diaphragmatic Hernia, Right-Sided Bochdalek

1. Cystic adenomatoid malformation (CAM) type III, sequestration, herniation of the liver into a diaphragmatic hernia in a right-sided Bochdalek hernia. Right-sided Bochdalek hernia. The curved arrow denotes the gallbladder.

2. Herniation of the liver above the right hemidiaphragm.

3. The portal vein.

4. Yes, the left lobe.

References

Guibaud L, Filiatrault D, Garel L, et al: Fetal congenital diaphragmatic hernia: Accuracy of sonography in the diagnosis and prediction of the outcome after birth. *AJR Am J Roentgenol* 166:1195–1202, 1996.

Hubbard AM, Adzick NS, Crombleholme TM, Haselgrove JC: Left-sided congenital diaphragmatic hernia: Value of prenatal MR imaging in preparation for fetal surgery. *Radiology* 203:636–640, 1997.

Cross-Reference
Ultrasound: THE REQUISITES, pp 245–246.

Comment

A left-sided congenital diaphragmatic hernia (CDH) is much more common than a right-sided (~7:1) hernia, and a right-sided CDH carries a worse prognosis. Bochdalek hernias are located laterally and more commonly on the left. Morgagni hernias are positioned medially, and the abdominal contents can herniate into the pericardium. The lateral and left-sided hernias are easier to detect with prenatal ultrasound than are the medial and right-sided ones.

It is important to try to determine the side of herniation. Fetal gallbladder (right-sided hernia) may be confused for the fetal stomach (left-sided hernia) (see Fig. B). In most right-sided CDHs, the stomach lies in its normal position. This case demonstrates a large right-sided hernia with the liver in the right hemithorax (see Figs. A to D). The left lobe of the liver can herniate into the left hemithorax with a left-sided diaphragmatic hernia. Magnetic resonance imaging (MRI) has been shown to be more accurate than ultrasound in confirming herniation of the liver.

Prenatal diagnosis is essential for counseling and surgical planning. The differential diagnosis includes other pulmonary masses, such as sequestration, bronchogenic cyst, and CAM. Because of the large cysts that can be seen with CAM type I, it can be more difficult to distinguish from the herniated bowel of a CDH. The paucity of abdominal structures aids in diagnosing CDH.

Notes

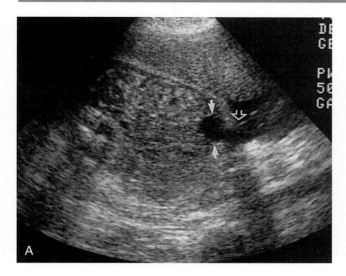

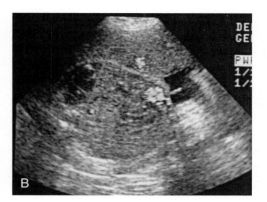

1. What finding (arrowheads) (Fig. A; open arrow = umbilical cord insertion) is detected anteriorly in the fetal abdomen of this second-trimester fetus? Figure B is a color Doppler image.

2. What is the normal caliber of the intra-abdominal portion of the umbilical vein?

3. Is this finding associated with other abnormalities?

4. Can Doppler imaging be valuable on follow-up examinations?

Umbilical Vein Varix

1. Umbilical vein varix.

2. The normal intra-abdominal umbilical vein measures 3 mm at 15 menstrual weeks and increases linearly to 8 mm at term.

3. Yes; there has been a reported association with third-trimester hydrops and fetal outcome.

4. Yes; it can evaluate the complication of varix thrombosis.

References

Dudiak CM, Salomon CG, Posniak HV, et al: Sonography of the umbilical cord. *Radiographics* 15:1035–1050, 1995.

Mahony BS, McGahan JP, Nyberg DA, Reisner DP: Varix of the fetal intra-abdominal umbilical vein: Comparison with normal. *J Ultrasound Med* 11:73–76, 1992.

White SP, Kofinas A: Prenatal diagnosis and management of umbilical vein varix of the intra-amniotic portion of the umbilical vein. *J Ultrasound Med* 13:992–994, 1994.

Cross-Reference

Ultrasound: THE REQUISITES, p 257.

Comment

The normal umbilical cord has two arteries and one vein. The single left umbilical vein, coursing with both umbilical arteries in the umbilical cord, joins the fetal left portal vein. It carries oxygenated blood to the fetus from the placenta. The umbilical arteries arise from the internal iliac arteries.

With ultrasound, the umbilical vein can be seen from its insertion at the anterior abdominal wall and can be followed into the liver on sagittal and oblique/transverse images. The normal size for the intra-abdominal extrahepatic portion of the umbilical vein is 3 mm at 15 weeks. The vein grows throughout the gestation to measure 8 mm at term. An umbilical vein varix is defined as a focal dilatation of the umbilical vein just inside the anterior abdominal wall (see Fig. A).

A varix more commonly involves the intra-amniotic portion (within the umbilical cord). The intra-amniotic varix can cause fetal demise due to thrombosis, and some recommend delivery as soon as lung maturity permits. An autopsy series has shown thrombosis of the varix to be a cause of stillbirth. An isolated intra-abdominal extrahepatic umbilical vein varix, which is demonstrated here, is rare. The literature is controversial with regard to its significance, and some report an increased risk of third-trimester hydrops and adverse fetal outcomes. The varicosity can thrombose and compromise delivery of oxygenated blood to the fetus.

Color Doppler imaging should be performed on all umbilical vein varicosities to document their patency, and close follow-up with serial ultrasound studies is advised.

The differential diagnosis of an intra-abdominal umbilical vein varix includes other cystic abdominal structures, such as the fetal gallbladder; a choledochal cyst; a mesenteric, ovarian, or urachal cyst; and a dilated bowel or genitourinary structure. Color Doppler imaging will document that the structure represents the umbilical vein varix, unless the varicosity has become thrombosed. Because of the risk of complications, some advocate delivery as soon as the fetal lungs mature.

Notes